As an expert in criminal tactics and personal security methods, Louis R. Mizell, Jr., has made numerous media appearances—including *The New York Times,* NBC Nightly News with Tom Brokaw, *The Philadelphia Inquirer,* and a variety of talk shows—to discuss ways that people can protect themselves from crime.

In *Street Sense for Women,* he offers specific, up-to-date advice on the techniques used by today's criminals and how to recognize and avoid dangerous situations—including such tactics as:

> *The "Good Samaritan" Ruse
> *The Unwitting Accomplice
> *Police Impersonation
> *The Postal Ploy
> *The Use of Classified Ads
> and more

Awareness is the key to saving lives, property, and money. This book will make you aware—and show you how to avoid becoming a victim.

STREET SENSE FOR WOMEN

How to Stay Safe in a Violent World

LOUIS R. MIZELL, JR.

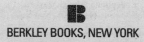

BERKLEY BOOKS, NEW YORK

STREET SENSE FOR WOMEN

A Berkley Book / published by arrangement with
the author

PRINTING HISTORY
Berkley edition / March 1993

ISBN: 0-425-13971-9

A BERKLEY BOOK® TM 757,375
Berkley Books are published by The Berkley Publishing Group,
200 Madison Avenue, New York, New York 10016.
The name "BERKLEY" and the "B" logo
are trademarks belonging to Berkley Publishing Corporation.

PRINTED IN THE UNITED STATES OF AMERICA

10 9 8 7 6 5 4 3

Dedicated with love
to my sister Jan
and to Leanna, Jamie, and Reed Smith

Contents

Acknowledgments

This important project for women is the result of a large group of professionals getting together as a team and making it happen. John Willig, my hard-charging literary agent, grabbed me by the collar and insisted that I get this data out of the computer and into a book, where it could do some good. The professional, winning team from Berkley Publishing—Karen Ravenel, Natalee Rosenstein, Donna Gould, Jacky Sach—the best of the best, were a pleasure to work with and won my deepest respect. A special thanks to Victoria Brown Barquero, my friend and associate, who wrestles daily with mountains of data and brings gentleness and genius, in five languages, to Mizell and Company. And a special thank you to my longtime gung-ho partner, Patrick (Eagle Eye) Friel, who personifies the warrior spirit, stood and fought, and didn't retreat an inch when the battle seemed lost. Enthusiastic about this book, there were a large number of wonderful, dedicated women who poured their time, support, and hearts into making this project a reality: Betty Baker, Shadia Barakat, Rebecca Boyd, Suzanne Conway, Anne Cusick, Laude Cuttier, Becky Frailey, Sally Hamilton, Aura Lippincott, Sheri Mestan, Mary Milewski, Esther Mizell, Karie Newmyer, Patty Raine, Penny Reid, Susan Stalick, Carol Stricker, Tammy Swankowski, Victoria Time. You are true professionals, loyal friends, and you are much appreciated. Keep smiling, stay positive, and stay safe.

Introduction

A petite, cheerful twenty-one-year-old woman left her New Jersey home August 21, 1992, to drive to college in Iowa. She was last seen looking under the hood of her car along Interstate 80 in Illinois and a long-haired trucker was apparently offering assistance. Her body, identified by dental records, was discovered nine days later, wrapped in a sheet, a red blanket, and duct tape. In Maryland, a thirty-four-year-old scientist, mother, and wife, was yanked from her BMW by two carjackers, November 8, 1992, and dragged one and a half miles to her death. During the ordeal, the carjackers tossed her baby daughter, still in the car seat, onto the road. In New York's Central Park a marauding pack of teenagers attacked a twenty-nine-year-old investment banker as she jogged alone past a grove of sycamore trees. For thirty minutes the boys gang-raped the five-foot-five, 100-pound Wellesley College graduate and brutally beat her with a brick, a rock, and a twelve-inch metal pipe. The "mindless marauders" gagged the woman with her

bloody shirt, fractured her skull, and left her naked
and unconscious in a mud puddle.

These three incidents symbolize the violence and
fear women must live with on a daily basis in our
society. Incredibly, nearly 20 million women were victims of rape, robbery, assault, murder, and a wide
range of other crimes in 1992. Every year tens of thousands of women are shot, stabbed, strangled, beaten,
or bludgeoned in the United States.

There are over 58,000 names on the Vietnam War
Memorial in Washington, D.C.; 58,000 names! But
during the next twenty-nine months more Americans,
women and men, will be murdered in the United
States than were killed in the entire Vietnam war.

The reality is that we live in a shockingly violent
society and street sense has become a necessity for
survival. The statistics are staggering. In the United
States during 1991 there were 24,703 murders; 106,593
reported rapes (12.1 million American women have
been the victim of forcible rape); 3,157,150 burglaries;
1,661,738 thefts of motor vehicles; 1,092,739 aggravated assaults; and 687,732 robberies. According
to the FBI Uniform Crime Report, these numbers
translate into one murder every 21 minutes, one rape
every 5 minutes, one burglary every 10 seconds, one
motor vehicle theft every 19 seconds, one aggravated
assault every 29 seconds, and one robbery every 46
seconds.

We are plagued with bullets, blood, and brutality,
and women are taking the brunt of the blow.

Although *Street Sense for Women* discusses dozens
of topics, the central theme, the thread running
throughout, concerns criminal deception. Criminals
use some form of deception, somewhere along the line,
in 90 percent of their operations; a trick, ruse, disguise, ploy, prop, or false story. Recognize the deception and *you* win. Fail to recognize the deception and

the *criminal* usually wins. Criminals use dozens of deceptive techniques to gain entry to your home and office, to set you up, to win your confidence, and to lure you into a trap.

Street Sense for Women chronicles the many tricks, ruses, and disguises used by serial murderers, robbers, rapists, burglars, bombers, kidnappers, con artists, child molesters, purse snatchers, and pickpockets. The more you know about criminal operations the better you will be at countering those operations. The tactics chronicled in this book are used against women in the street, and in offices, hotels, homes, airports, and shopping malls. The different chapters will also show how thousands of women are being attacked in their driveways, at automatic teller machines (ATMs), and pay telephones.

In the chapter on carjackings you will learn about the "bump and rob" technique, the "follow home" tactic, the good samaritan ruse, the valet parking tricks, and much, much more. In the chapter on pickpockets and bag snatchers you will learn the distractions and tricks criminals have used to steal thousands of purses, briefcases, and wallets: the crumpled money trick, the ketchup squirt, the baby bounce, and the escalator dance.

A wide variety of criminals from pickpockets to serial murderers have posed as police, postmen, plumbers, and photographers.

Deception takes many forms. To appear helpless and harmless, serial murderer Ted Bundy wore a cast, faked a broken arm, and then asked women for assistance. To surveil a neighborhood one burglar jogged the streets, another pretended to be walking his dog, and a criminal couple, looking for open garages, innocently pushed a baby carriage. In New York, a transient donned a stethoscope and white lab coat and "became" a doctor in a major hospital. He raped and murdered a female doctor working alone.

To appear innocent and non-threatening, criminals have worked as couples walking arm in arm, looking lovingly into each other's eyes. Criminals can be very old and very young; they have posed as priests, nuns, and rabbis; and in thirty cases known to the author, rapists, robbers, and other criminals feigned the need for a wheelchair. To create the image of sweetness and vulnerability some female street criminals have even used pillows as props and become instantly pregnant. All is not always as it appears to be.

Utilizing a repertoire of disguises and diversions, ploys and props, false stories and false identifications, today's criminals are truly masters of deception.

It is important that we understand the domino, cause-and-effect aspects of crime. One woman, thinking crime only happens in "bad" neighborhoods, left her purse on the front seat of her car, a security mistake. A thief smashed her window and stole her purse. Using the keys in the purse, the thief burglarized the woman's home and tied and raped her thirteen-year-old daughter who had been sleeping. Finding the woman's ATM code number in a pile of personal papers, the thief then emptied her bank account.

In this age of violence, one person's mistake can affect us all. A person falls for a sad story, carries someone else's "duty free" bottles on to an airplane, and 300 people are at risk if those bottles are booby-trapped. A sorority sister whines, "Locking doors is such a hassle," and five of her friends could be bludgeoned to death. If a hotel or apartment manager is careless with the passkey (as so frequently happens) a woman could be, and often is, raped, robbed, or murdered.

It's important to know that some serial murderers and rapists respond to your classified ads (Stereo for

Sale), bringing them to you. And other serial murderers and rapists place their own ads (Jewelry for Sale), hoping to lure you to them.

And it is important to know that in literally thousands of cases, a collection of con artists, kidnappers, rapists, and robbers have preceded their crime with one of three questions: "May I use your telephone?", "Do you have the time?", and (asking directions) "Can you tell me how I get to . . . ?"

In any human endeavor, attitude is extremely important, and this is especially true for security. Don't think, "It can't happen to me or my loved ones." Millions of people live their lives as if it won't happen to them and millions of people each year are wide-eyed with shock when it does happen to them. Don't think security is someone else's job. Wake up! Security is *your* job, no one else can look after you. "Oh, I'm not worried about myself." If that's the way you feel, fine. But please make sure your complacency, your lack of security, doesn't get someone else hurt. "Well, if they want to get you, they're going to get you." Nonsense! That's the worse attitude of all! You don't let them get you. Period. "Oh, I grew up in New York, I know just about everything there is to know about security." No, you don't! There's more to learn and the more you know the safer you are. Knowledge is power. You don't have to say, "If I had only known . . ."

Although this book is about knowledge, not karate, you need to develop your own philosophy concerning fighting. Most experts will tell you "never resist," and in most cases they will be right. But in the real world we all know there is a time when you have to resist, you have to fight for survival. But no book, no expert can make that decision for you. There are too many variables, too many different situations, and too many criminal personalities. When you are being dragged into the bushes, when your child is threatened, you are on your own. The experts are home watching television.

There are thousands of cases in which women have screamed, resisted, run, punched, kicked, and saved themselves, and, unfortunately, there are thousands of cases in which the same behavior made things worse. There are success stories and sad stories. One woman screamed and scared her assailant; one woman screamed and was slashed for doing so. One woman struck her assailant and was saved, another struck her assailant and was shot. Clearly, your decision to fight should be based on survival, not anger, not ego. Your decision should be based on reason, not panic. You do not risk it all for a purse. Remember, many muggers do not display a weapon until they meet with resistance and many purse snatchers who appear to be alone and unarmed work with armed backups or lookouts.

If you come home and see a burglar in your house you'd be a fool to charge in out of anger. Don't fight in that case. Keep a distance and call the police.

Yes, in the real world there is a time to fight but that decision can only be made by you. But if you fight you "go animal" and you fight to win; no squeamishness, no mercy allowed. You bite and rip a nose, a neck, anything you come in contact with. You viciously claw an eye, you kick, knee, and grab a groin aggressively. And remember, if your instincts tell you to "go for it" you are ten times stronger and more vicious than you ever imagined. You can win, you can survive.

Your fight/flight philosophy should also be discussed with your mate and your sons. Chivalry is not dead and many men, if threatened, will fight on impulse, partly out of instinct and partly because they feel that you (the woman) expect it! Therefore, it is

important to discuss with your husband/boyfriend/
son your fight/flight philosophy. If you do not want
them to risk it all for a purse or a home burglary, tell
them so!

There is a phenomenon, a security disease if you
will, called "magical thinking." Too many of us suffer
from this disease. "I don't worry about locking my
door in the daytime." Fact: Sixty percent of burglaries
occur in the daylight hours. Tens of thousands of
rapes and other crimes have occurred in homes during
the day. "I don't worry about locking the doors when
my husband is home." Fact: In 1991 approximately
480,000 homes were entered by criminals while at least
one member of the family was present in the house. At
least 144,000 of these burglaries resulted in at least one
family member being murdered, wounded, raped, or
violently attacked. "I don't lock my doors when my
husband is home." Great! Don't you realize husbands
get killed, too! Lock your doors! "This is a safe neighborhood, we've never had a crime problem." Wake
up! First, you'd be amazed at how many crimes have
occurred in your neighborhood! Just because you
don't know about them, it doesn't mean they didn't
occur. Second, for every rape victim, every carjacking
victim, every shooting victim, there was a time when
they reasoned (magical thinking) that "Since this has
not happened to me in the past it won't happen to me
in the future." There's always a first time and when
that first time happens to you, you are sorry, very
sorry, you didn't practice better security. There are no
safe neighborhoods!

"I'm pretty good about locking my car doors when
I'm in town." Lock your car doors all the time! Fact:
Thousands of carjackings, robberies, rapes, kidnappings, and other crimes would be prevented each year
if people would wise up and lock their car doors.

Thousands of crimes occur in private driveways. Get the facts and examine your "magical thinking."

Street Sense for Women is designed to help save lives, property, and money. The crime problem is real and it's here to stay. You will be targeted. But you do not have to be a victim. You do not have to say, "If I had only known . . ."

1

Stage Props

Just as stage actors and magicians use props to divert attention or to create an illusion, criminal conjurers do the same thing.

In New York City a transient put a stethoscope around his neck and, "abracadabra," he became a doctor in a major hospital. The transient roamed the halls until he spotted a woman doctor working alone in her office. The doctor was raped and murdered. Employees who saw the man walking the halls admitted they didn't recognize him but stated that he looked like a doctor. The employees were lulled into complacency with a prop, a prop that has been used by hundreds of criminals inside and outside the medical environment.

A man who stole purses and other valuables from high-rise office buildings told the author he never went to "work" without his insect extermination equipment. "Sometimes I'd tell all the secretaries they would have to leave while I fumigated the offices," he said. Of course, when the secretaries left the office the

1

"exterminator" was free to rifle drawers, closets, and purses. "No one was suspicious of my mask because they thought it was to protect me from the fumes," he said. The office thief further explained that most of the stolen merchandise was hidden in the false bottom of the spray canister. For the purposes of this thief, the insect exterminator props were perfect.

Ted Bundy, who raped and murdered many women in the United States, used fake casts and splints as props and pretended to have a broken arm or leg. In one case he is believed to have targeted a woman leaving a library. Wearing a splint on one hand and a sling on the opposite arm, Bundy dropped a load of books and, for effect, grimaced in pain. Predictably, the concerned woman probably asked: "Do you need some assistance?" Without suspecting what was in store for her, the woman is believed to have helped Bundy carry his books to a dark and isolated area where he parked his car.

At a lakeside recreational area, Bundy, with one arm in a sling, approached women and asked if they would be so kind as to help him lower his sailboat from his car. His car, of course, was parked in a deserted, wooded area. In other cases Bundy hobbled along on crutches and a fake leg cast and solicited help in carrying his briefcase. Bundy was a master of the physical disability ruse and used it fatally. He was, after all, a polite, good-looking young man who seemed harmless because of his handicaps. He could not possibly be the monster police were looking for.

Setting the stage with props, psychology, and persona, today's criminal actor masks his true self and pretends to be an innocent part of the scenery.

A thief using paint buckets and brushes as props breezed through an apartment complex in Washington, D.C., magically making jewelry and other valuables mysteriously disappear. Twelve tenants were asked if they had seen anyone suspicious in the complex and all twelve responded no. When asked if they had seen a painter on the premises, most of the same tenants responded yes. None of the dozen witnesses, however, had actually seen any painting being done. The thief's props served two purposes. To some, this "workman" was a non-person, an invisible human being. To others, the props communicated that he belonged, that he was okay. He could not possibly be the thief. He could not possibly be the man who raped two women in their apartments. But the evidence and the jury say differently.

It is not enough to "look for anything suspicious" because in most cases it's not the "suspicious" we are looking for, but that which appears absolutely innocent.

In crime, as in magic, all is not always as it appears to be. Exploiting our personal perceptions and prejudices, a parade of rapists, robbers, muggers, and murderers have marched invisibly into apartment complexes, office buildings, and government installations.

Although many of the props being used against women are quite imaginative, a cast of crusaders, criminals, and crazies are also utilizing props that are quite simple, but effective.

One rapist carried a clipboard and stuffed his shirt pockets full of pens. He'd write while he walked, take a few notes on his clipboard, and check the hallway for unlocked doors. Another robber/rapist carried a bucket and mop as props but he was not the type to work for a living.

Props are utilized in all aspects of crime against women. A prop can be used to surveil a neighborhood or to conceal weapons and stolen merchandise. A criminal may use a prop that communicates "I am innocent, harmless, and non-threatening." Props are used by burglars, bombers, swindlers, and smugglers.

A burglar surveilled a neighborhood walking his dog. The dog prop made people think he belonged, he had a purpose for being in the neighborhood. Numerous criminal couples and female offenders have pushed a baby buggy to appear non-threatening as they walked a neighborhood looking for prime targets. To create an image of sweetness and vulnerability, several female terrorists and street criminals have used pillows as props and become instantly pregnant. In Connecticut, one burglar used a basketball as a prop to appear nonchalant. When he would set off a burglar alarm, he would casually bounce the basketball down the street as police cars whizzed by.

Some form of deception is used in 90 percent of the attacks on women: a prop, a ruse, a disguise, a false story, etc. Recognize the deception and you win. Fail to recognize the deception, the illusion, and the criminal wins.

A wide range of criminals and crazies have accomplished their deeds using religious props. A pickpocket put people at ease and subtly communicated that he was honest by carrying a Bible. A burglar in a Jewish community wore a yarmulke.

Flowers are frequently used as props. In fact, some of the unkindest cuts of all have been delivered with a beautiful bouquet of flowers. As a ploy to gain entry, conceal a bomb, or drop the guard of their victims, a wide range of people—mafia hitmen, political extremists, robbers, and even jealous lovers—have accomplished their criminal intentions under the pretext of delivering flowers.

Traditionally, lovers give flowers to one another as a sign of affection. On occasion, however, when love turns to hate, the delivery of flowers takes on a new meaning. On February 26, 1986, a twenty-five-year-old Virginia woman attacked her ex-boyfriend's fiancée after disguising herself as a flower delivery person. She painted on a mustache, donned a delivery cap, and rang the doorbell at her former boyfriend's home. When the fiancée answered the door, the assailant announced, "Flower delivery," and then slashed at the victim with a seven-inch knife.

On November 18, 1986, a man donned a white tuxedo, a wig, and false beard and delivered a booby-trapped bouquet to a government building in San Francisco. The bomb hidden in the flowers exploded and injured two women. One of them was the estranged wife of the millionaire who had plotted the bombing. She had filed for divorce and was seeking a large settlement.

Should you be more suspicious of a man carrying a paint bucket or a woman pushing a baby buggy or a person with a broken leg or a bouquet of flowers? Of course not! The point is that you can't be *less* suspicious.

A magician can perform a trick and you are amazed. How did he do that? You don't see the illusion, the deception. But if the same magician takes you aside and explains in detail how the trick is managed, you are no longer fooled. Now, looking at the same trick, it's easy to see how he does it. The magic is gone. Well, it's up to you to take the magic away from the criminals.

REDUCING THE RISK

1. Don't become cynical but develop a healthy sense of suspicion and a good eye for deception.

2. Realize that in the real world there is some evil and a lot of violence. Realize that in the real world you need street sense for survival.

3. All is not always as it appears to be. Get involved in crime prevention, ask questions, report situations you think might be dangerous. Remember the "exterminator"? Well, he went into nearly 200 offices and nobody ever asked, "Who sent for him?" Nobody ever asked, "Why do I have to leave my office?" Nobody ever thought, Hey, this guy could be stealing purses. Remember the painter? He was seen in the building eight times but nobody ever saw him paint! Remember the dog walker? *After* a rash of burglaries a woman said, "I thought it was odd that he'd drive to this neighborhood, walk his dog, and then drive away. . . . I wish I had gotten his license plate number."

4. Don't be lulled into complacency because of a prop. If you wouldn't normally escort a stranger to a dark, isolated area, then don't escort a man just because he has a cast on his leg. If you don't normally leave your purse unattended on a train when you use the rest room, then don't leave it unattended just because the person next to you is reading the Bible.

5. Remember, a prop can be a camera (see "Phony Photographers and the Modeling Masquerade"), a crucifix, a basketball, a baby buggy, a clipboard, or a pocket full of pens.

6. Don't let the criminals have all the fun! You can use props, too. You don't have a guard dog? Put a huge dog dinner bowl on your front porch. If you like inscribe the dog's name on the bowl, e.g., "Dobby the Doberman" or "Mr. Peter Pit Bull." You don't have a burglar alarm? Hey, there's

nothing stopping you from buying a burglar alarm decal for your home or car. Be creative, show some street sense, and use all the weapons at your disposal to avoid being a victim.

2
Carjackings

The Maryland scientist certainly never imagined her life would be ended by a carjacker. But on November 8, 1992, in a peaceful, middle-class neighborhood, she was yanked out of her car by two carjackers and dragged one and a half miles to her death. It was eight-thirty in the morning and she was driving her baby daughter to daycare. When she stopped at a stop sign, two men apparently opened her unlocked door, pulled her out, and drove off with her daughter still strapped in her car seat. Probably snagged on the seat belt, the victim was seen being dragged beside the car at a high rate of speed. After the carjackers drove a short distance, they stopped the car and tossed the baby, still in the car seat, onto the road. Then, with a squeal of tires, the carjackers continued on and tried to dislodge the woman from the side of her BMW by sideswiping a fence. Within hours police had arrested the two men, who had dragged a woman to her death and discarded a baby like litter, just to steal an automobile.

Nearly 1.7 million vehicles are stolen each year in the United States (one car stolen approximately every nineteen seconds), and in 1992 an estimated 28,000 of these vehicles were stolen by armed carjackers. Unlike ordinary car thieves who steal parked, unattended vehicles, "carjackers" attack while the driver and passengers are in or near the vehicle. The ordinary car thief has to break into the vehicle and either "hotwire" the engine or target people who have left the keys in the ignition. The carjacker, however, simply puts a gun to the driver's head; demands the keys, purses, and wallets; and drives away.

To date, thousands of women in the United States have lost their vehicles to carjackers and hundreds of these women have also been murdered, injured, kidnapped, or raped.

In upper-class Bethesda, Maryland, a forty-five-year-old university professor was shot and killed for her car outside the National Institute of Health. Gunmen in Michigan forced a Suzuki Sidekick to the curb, shouted, "Gimme your car, bitch," and murdered the woman driver. In Piscataway, New Jersey, November 3, 1992, a mother left her home at seven-thirty P.M. to run errands with her three-year-old daughter. Her husband stayed home with their two other children. The woman had just returned a video and was stopped at a red light when a man leaped into her apparently unlocked 1992 Plymouth van. The three-year-old was found shivering and confused at six-thirty the next morning. The victim's naked and stabbed body was discovered in a drainage ditch four days later.

As these cases so graphically illustrate, when a carjacker steals a car, anything in that car, including children, goes with him. In fact, carjackers and ordinary car thieves have abducted at least twenty children in recent years.

Although we should be careful not to blame the

victim—the criminal is to blame—hundreds of car-jackings would have been prevented if the victim had simply locked the car doors. These preventable car-jackings include many cases that endangered children.

While sitting in her car one hot Sunday afternoon, a New Jersey woman, waiting to make a turn, reached over and tried to coax a giggle out of her baby girl. Without warning, a man opened her door and started pulling her from the car. As reported in the *New York Times,* she screamed, "Take the car, but let me have my baby!" The carjacker, however, sped off as she clung to a leather strap. She was dragged fifteen yards before her grip gave way. Fortunately, after a night of terror for the family, the baby was discovered in the car, which was abandoned. She was crying and dehydrated, but otherwise unharmed.

Many infants and small children have also been abducted from parked vehicles while parents and baby-sitters were making a quick telephone call, buying a newspaper, or using an automatic teller machine (ATM). People rationalize that they will only be gone a minute, so they leave the keys in the ignition and the engine running. And time and again carjackers have exploited this "one minute" and stolen cars with small children in the backseat.

In Dallas, Texas, a young mother parked her car in front of a grocery store, left the engine running, and told her two little boys to lock the door behind her. They failed to do so. While she was in the store a man jumped in the car and took off with the children. Fortunately, a massive police search discovered the boys two hours later. The thief had dumped the children in a park. Since the temperatures were below freezing, the boys were cold and scared but, happily, unhurt.

A car thief in Elgin, Illinois, also drove away with more than he had bargained for. A woman pulled up to a grocery store and left her four-year-old daughter asleep on the front seat, and the car's engine running. When the woman returned with her groceries her car and daughter were gone. An hour later, the longest hour in this mother's life, the police received an anonymous call and were told where they could find the little girl. Although frightened, the little girl was unharmed.

Carjackers and ordinary car thieves have been very young and very old: eight years old to eighty years old. They have been shabbily dressed and attired in tailored business suits. Sometimes they work alone and sometimes they work in teams. Sometimes the carjackers work as a male-and-female couple and sometimes carjackers have utilized children as props, to win your confidence. In over 100 cases reported to the author, the carjackers have been *female*.

In Philadelphia, a twenty-three-year-old woman stole a car and an eighteen-month-old boy who was asleep in that car. The child's mother left the car's engine running and went into a post office to mail some letters. Another woman stole a car and a fourteen-month-old baby in Prince George's County, Maryland. The child's father parked his car outside a repair shop and stepped inside to talk with the mechanic. Within one minute, the female carjacker jumped into the vehicle and drove away. On November 14, 1992, in Camden, New Jersey, a woman pointed a handgun through a car window and screamed to the driver, "Get out, now!" When the driver got out, the woman got in and drove away. A month earlier in Michigan, a forty-three-year-old woman shot a police officer and stole his patrol car. Do not underestimate the female criminal!

Some female carjackers are stealing cars even though they are not old enough to drive. In September 1992, police in Washington, D.C., arrested two girls,

ages fourteen and fifteen, and charged them with carjacking. The girls approached a man driving a 1987
Honda, pointed a nine-millimeter semi-automatic
handgun at his head, and screamed in high pitched
voices, "Gimme you car."

One of the most popular tactics used by carjackers
and other highway criminals is the "bump and rob"
technique. Using the "bump and rob" tactic, the criminal feigns an accident by bumping into your back
bumper. You get out to inspect the damage and your
car is stolen or you may be robbed, raped, or kidnapped. In 1992, versions of the "bump and rob"
tactic victimized over 3,000 people in the United
States.

In Michigan, a forty-year-old woman was driving a
1989 Cougar when she was struck from behind. When
the woman got out to check the damage, a man with
a handgun took her car and purse. The gunman fired
a shot at the woman when she ran to a nearby house.

A twenty-six-year-old California woman was returning home from the airport when another car rear-
ended her. She followed the other car to a dark side
street until it stopped. When she got out to inspect
the damage the men stole her car and her young daughter,
who was asleep on the backseat. Dumped out of the
car, the girl was recovered seven long hours later,
when she wandered into a stranger's yard and cried,
"I've been kidnapped."

Another tactic growing in popularity is the so-called
good samaritan tactic. There are several versions of
the good samaritan tactic. In Maryland a clean-cut,
polite, and well-dressed man stole twenty-one cars,
mostly from women. This man would point to the
back of a motorist's vehicle and warn them about a
(non-existent) wobbly wheel or flaming exhaust. He
would point and say, "Ma'am, you're losing your left
rear wheel." The woman would get out of her car to

inspect the problem and the "good samaritan" would jump in and drive away.

On the Baltimore-Washington Parkway in Maryland a good samaritan helped fix a woman's car that had broken down. Once he got the car running, he pulled a weapon and stole it. (It's quite possible the man sabotaged the vehicle in the first place.)

Another carjacker in Maryland feigned an injury and flagged down a man and wife who were driving a Jeep. The couple asked the man, "What's the matter?" He pulled a gun and responded, "I need your car."

Good samaritans around the country have developed a technique that produces a slow leak in a motorist's tire. The criminals simply follow the target, and when her tire goes flat on the interstate, they rush in and rob or rape the woman. This tactic has most frequently been used against jewelry salespersons and people transporting payrolls.

Women should be very suspicious of men who magically appear when they have a flat tire. There are many recorded cases of rapists and serial murderers who flatten women's tires or sabotage their engines in a parking lot and then show up and offer a lift.

Increasingly, carjackers and a wide variety of other criminals are utilizing the "follow home" tactic. Following their target from a shopping center, grocery store, ATM, etc., the criminals frequently attack the motorist in her own driveway. Thousands of women have been victimized by the "follow home" tactic.

A man dubbed the "carjacking king" by Detroit police was arrested in 1991 and believed to be responsible for fifty-four carjackings. In a newspaper interview, he stated he would follow his victims "for miles." "Once they got where they were going, then I'd take the car," he said. "If people had been more observant, saw me following them, and drove to a police station, then I would have driven off."

In addition to the "bump and rob," "good samaritan," and "follow home" techniques a wide range of male and female carjackers, young and old, are continuously devising creative new ways to steal your vehicle.

One particularly novel technique that has been reported in several states is the "valet parking" ruse. In some cases, thieves have staked out fancy restaurants that have a valet parking service and a clientele likely to drive expensive cars. When the restaurant parking attendant leaves to park one vehicle, the carjacker quickly takes his place and pretends to be another parking attendant. When another customer drives her car up, the thief smiles, graciously opens the door, says, "Thank you, ma'am" for the tip . . . and parks the car in another city. After dinner, when the owner tries to claim her Mercedes, the real valet, looking confused, says, "What Mercedes?"

As the most violent new crime of the 1990s, carjacking incidents are in the headlines almost every day. But the cases that are rarely publicized are the victories: hundreds of incidents in which motorists have thwarted attempted carjackings.

On the morning of September 15, 1992, in Baltimore, Maryland, an armed man ordered a thirty-two-year-old woman out of her car as she waited at a red light. Instead, she stepped on the gas and speeded through the intersection. She stopped a mile up the road and called police but the gunman had vanished by the time officers arrived.

Many women, seeing armed men approach their cars at intersections, have stepped on the gas and escaped. Dozens of women have reported cases in which men have attempted, unsuccessfully, to open their locked car doors. One woman, at a self-service gas station, saw a man jump into her car when she walked over to pay the cashier. Since the woman had taken the keys out of the ignition, the same man quickly jumped out of the car and fled. Savvy to the "bump and rob" tactic, a woman in Florida, who was rear-ended at one A.M., drove slowly to a safe area before pulling over. The other driver took off, but the woman got his license plate number. His car had been reported stolen.

One success story that did receive a lot of publicity was the case of a senior-citizen widow who foiled an attempt to steal her sporty 1991 Nissan Maxima. On November 26, 1992, the feisty widow was driving on Long Island when two men stopped their car in front of her so that she could not pass. One of the men ran back to her car, banged on the window, and ordered her to get out. Instead, she put the car in reverse, and the man ran back to his car. Giving chase, the men tried to ram their vehicle into hers, but she avoided a collision by driving onto the sidewalk and over lawns. At one point during the chase the men sideswiped her car, and the woman, in a scene reminiscent of the chariot race in *Ben Hur,* sideswiped the men. Banging off each other from side to side, the men were eventually able to pull in front and again block her forward movement. This time when the man ran back, the widow put her car in drive and tried to "run him down and kill him." She missed. But when the man grabbed her steering wheel through the window, she floored her car in reverse and dragged the man until he was forced to let go. The two men then fled. Quoted in a newspaper, she said, "I hope I scared the ——— out of them so they never try another carjacking again. I think they were carjacking virgins."

In the battle against carjackers, some women have screamed and scared off the attacker; some women have screamed and been shot. On August 28, 1992, in

Maryland in broad daylight a young woman was approached by a gunman in the parking lot of a shopping center. The gunman grabbed the woman roughly, pointed a gun at her, and demanded the keys to her sports car. She refused, pulled away, and started screaming. The man got scared and ran away. The woman was lucky. She only suffered a torn dress and a bloody lip.

Another woman in a similar situation was not so lucky. In New Jersey, October 19, 1992, at five P.M., a middle-aged woman was approached by a carjacker in a supermarket parking lot. As she was getting out of her 1981 car, the gunman appeared and ordered her to move over. The woman screamed and the man shot her in the leg at point-blank range. The woman fell from the car bleeding profusely and the man jumped in her car and drove off.

The violent carjacking trend will certainly continue through the 1990s. Women and men will continue to be targeted while they are using pay telephones, ATMs, and while they are pumping gas at self-service gas stations. Armed carjackings will also occur in office parking lots, shopping malls, car washes, and while victims are stopped at traffic lights. This is the reality. The solution is to dramatically reduce the risk by becoming street smart.

REDUCING THE RISK

1. Keep your car door locked at all times. When slowed in traffic or stopped at a traffic light, it is better to keep your windows at least three-fourths of the way up. Thousands of carjackings and other crimes would have been prevented if the car doors had been locked!

2. When pumping gas, using a telephone, or leaving your car for any reason take your keys with you. We are making it too easy for the criminals. Over 200,000 vehicles are stolen each year in the United States because the driver left the keys in the ignition! Don't leave your keys in the car, not even for one minute.

3. Be alert, be aware of surroundings. When you are stopped, parking, or moving slowly, look around. Watch for suspicious activity or innocent behavior that could turn dangerous. What is your escape route? Be ready to drive on. When stopped, don't read, put on lipstick, or comb your hair. There are more important things to attend to.

4. At a stoplight or when traffic is moving slowly, keep a distance between you and the car in front of you. If possible, don't box yourself in. This will allow you room to maneuver in an emergency. Don't be afraid to use your horn to attract attention to yourself or your would-be attacker. Noise is a great deterrent to crime.

5. Buy gas during the day at a location you consider relatively safe. Remember, in this age of violence many women have paid dearly for running out of gas at the wrong place and the wrong time.

6. Don't park in secluded or poorly lighted places at night.

7. If you are walking to your car and see (or sense) someone moving with you or loitering near your vehicle, walk away and observe. If the situation

disturbs you, ask for assistance or call the police. Be very suspicious of someone who magically appears and offers you a ride when you have a flat tire.

8. If you think someone is following your vehicle, drive to a police station or drive to a safe, populated area and call police. Be especially suspicious if you see the same car at different times or on different days. The cold facts are that tens of thousands of crime victims in the United States were followed from the interstate or from the home, office, shopping centers, etc. Be observant!

9. If an armed person demands your keys or your car you are statistically better off if you do not resist. Yes, many have resisted and won, but many more have resisted and ended up maimed, paralyzed, or dead. Remember, the battle isn't over yet; there's a good chance your information or someone else's information will put the criminal in jail.

10. If you are uncomfortable about someone approaching your car, don't stop to think what they want. Quickly determine a safe escape route and *drive.* Listen to your instincts.

11. Remember, the carjackers have been old and young, male and female, black and white. Carjackers have been well dressed and poorly dressed; they have operated as man and wife and have used children as props to put you at ease. They steal expensive cars and they steal old economy models. In New Orleans (1991), a polite, well-dressed man and wife told a thirty-year-old

woman that their car had broken down and they needed a lift. The "wife" held a baby in her arms. When the couple got in the woman's car, they pulled weapons and demanded her belongings. The couple then tied and gagged the woman and kept her hostage in the trunk of her car for twenty-four hours.

12. Over 3,000 people were victimized by the "bump and rob" tactic in 1992. Don't get paranoid (most accidents are legitimate), but if you are rear-ended with minor damage, drive to a safe, well-lighted area before exiting your vehicle. Realizing that all is not always as it appears to be, assess your own situation and determine if you consider the situation suspicious and/or dangerous.

13. Be alert to the good samaritan ruses and other schemes designed to lure you out of your car. Ask yourself, How vulnerable am I if I get out of my car? If someone points to your "wobbly back tire" you might want to wave, say thank you, and drive a block before inspecting it. In Silver Spring, Maryland, on August 12, 1992, a carjacker, pretending to be a good samaritan, stole a woman's BMW after pointing out damage from an alleged hit and run. The forty-year-old woman had just climbed into her car when the man tapped on her window and explained that he had seen someone hit her car. When the woman got out to inspect the damage, the man pulled a handgun and stole the BMW.

14. Do not leave children in an unattended vehicle with the keys in the ignition. (Although one mother kiddingly said this would be a great way

to punish carjackers!) The author knows of more than twenty children abducted accidentally by carjackers. If you must leave children in the car unattended for a few minutes, (a) do not leave the engine running, (b) do not leave the keys in the ignition, and (c) do not leave the doors unlocked.

15. In winter stay with your vehicle while you are warming it up. Many people start the engine and go back inside the house while the car warms up. Carjackers appreciate this very much.

16. Don't keep your car keys with your house and office keys. If they steal your car keys you don't want them having access to your home and office. Besides, if your car is stolen you'll be in no mood to be locked out of your own home! Using keys and information found in stolen vehicles, carjackers have frequently committed many additional crimes.

17. Many women have been dragged by their own vehicles after being carjacked. If you are pulled or ordered from your car, step clear of the door and make sure you are not entangled with your seat belt; make sure your coat, scarf, and other clothing do not get caught in the doors.

18. Be sure you know who you are giving your car keys to; car thieves have posed as parking attendants at garages and restaurants.

19. Thousands of victims have been locked in their own trunks by a wide variety of criminals. High-profile or high-threat citizens may want to invest in an inside latch for their trunk. Many locksmiths can rig a release device for you.

20. Do not rent vehicles that are clearly marked as rental vehicles. Thieves often target rentals because they believe they are driven by tourists who carry a lot of money. The criminal also knows that most tourists won't return for a court case.

21. If you leave packages, purses, and briefcases in view on the car seats, there's a good chance a criminal will smash a window and grab your valuables. Remember "smash and grabs" occur when the car is parked *and* when it is being driven.

22. Be aware of diversions and distractions. Often one criminal will try to sell something to the driver while a second criminal enters the car or steals a purse from the passenger side of the vehicle.

23. In many foreign countries, and to a lesser extent in the United States, criminals will throw something in your car window (a burning piece of paper, a live rat) in hopes you will jump out of your car. When you jump out, the criminal either robs you or steals your car.

24. In many countries criminals surveil parking lots and watch where you put your car keys (in your purse, in your left pocket, etc.). Perhaps one mile from the parking lot the criminal snatches your purse and then runs back to the car he saw you exit. Protect your car keys. A simple purse snatching can lead to a car theft.

25. Remember, thousands of people in the United States have been attacked, robbed, raped, kid-

napped, or murdered in their own driveways. And this trend is increasing!

26. Car alarms and security devices that lock the steering wheel in place are a good idea for parked vehicles. (The irony is that these devices have been so effective they have probably contributed to the increase in armed carjackings from drivers.) Security companies can also provide fuel and ignition shut-off switches and even electronic tracking devices that allow your car to be located if stolen.

27. Car phones are an excellent security idea, providing they do not hinder your concentration while driving.

28. Warning: Many vehicles, advertised for sale by the owners, have been stolen when a prospective buyer took the car for a test drive.

29. Keep your cool in traffic. Many motorists have been shot simply for screaming at another driver or for raising a middle finger in the well-known sign of disgust. If you exit your vehicle to give another driver a piece of your mind you risk life and limb.

30. Be a survivor: be street smart.

3

Automatic Teller Machines (ATMs)

A New York doctor had just withdrawn fifty dollars from a bank automatic teller machine (ATM) when two men jumped into her unlocked luxury car. With a gun pointed at her head, she was forced to drive her car to Brooklyn, where she was beaten to death after refusing to give her abductors her personal identification number (PIN).

The doctor is just one of thousands of women to be victimized by an ATM-related crime. And like her, many of these women have suffered more than just a loss of money; they have been kidnapped, raped, and even murdered.

ATMs have definitely become a criminal's dream and a customer's security nightmare. State senator Charles M. Calderon, a crusader for better ATM security, was quoted in the *Los Angeles Times* as saying, "It is the crime of the nineties . . . the problem is much worse than we've ever imagined." The senator's statement followed several highly publicized ATM incidents. A California woman was abducted from an

ATM, raped, and shot in the head. A twenty-two-year-old woman in Alabama was abducted from an ATM, robbed, murdered, and set on fire. A woman in Illinois was forced to withdraw four hundred dollars from an ATM and then murdered by her abductors.

One of the biggest complaints from women victimized at ATMs has been lack of security. A widow of a man murdered during an ATM robbery alleges that she and her husband were robbed because the bank had failed to provide adequate lighting at its cash machine and had located the ATM away from the public view. The woman, who has filed a multimillion-dollar wrongful death lawsuit against the bank has complained that all the normal safeguards—lighting, video cameras, security guards, panic buttons, etc.— were absent when her husband was robbed of forty dollars and she was robbed of her husband.

A Washington, D.C., woman also complains of inadequate ATM security. She was on her way to the beach one morning when she decided to stop at a bank ATM, located blocks from the Capitol. As she entered her PIN a man came up behind her, put his arm around her waist, displayed a handgun, and demanded that she take out three hundred dollars. She noted that the robber had no problem following her into the premises because the lock on the door was broken. No one could see her being robbed because the windows were tinted to keep the area cooler. A bank security camera recorded the robbery but, as so frequently happens, the poor quality of equipment rendered the tape useless. Finally, the woman told the author that an armed security guard witnessed the entire robbery but his actions or inactions may have actually endangered her life. Instead of calling police or taking other appropriate actions, the security guard attempted to remotely turn off the ATM. In his haste, he turned off the wrong machine. She speculates that if her machine had failed to produce the three hundred dollars, the nervous gunman may have blamed her and started shooting.

But not all ATM-related crimes can be blamed on inadequate physical security at ATM facilities. Sometimes careless "personal security" contributes to ATM-related crimes.

In one case a woman left her purse on the front seat of her car, a security mistake. A drug addict smashed the car window and stole the purse containing her house keys. Using the keys, the man burglarized the woman's house and discovered her PIN in a pile of personal papers. Using the stolen bank card and PIN, the man made five ATM withdrawals.

In another case, at 2:15 in the afternoon, two men simply walked in the unlocked front door of a private residence in Germantown, Maryland, and pulled guns on the residents, a wife and husband in their fifties. The gunmen stole valuables from the home and drove the couple to an ATM, where they were forced to make sizable withdrawals.

And sometimes inadequate security at apartment buildings, offices, shopping centers, and so forth also contributes to ATM-related crimes.

A young woman had just walked into the unsecured lobby of her Chicago apartment building and was collecting her mail when four armed men approached her and forced her outside. Concerns about inadequate access controls in the building had apparently fallen on deaf ears. The men took her to an ATM and ordered her to withdraw four hundred dollars. After receiving the money, the men marched the young woman into an alley and murdered her with a shot to the head.

Step one in any effective security program is to identify the problem and face up to reality, no matter how frightening. And the reality of the ATM issue is that a Washington, D.C., woman was abducted by two men, forced to withdraw two hundred dollars from an ATM, and then strangled to death. The reality is that a woman in Toronto, Canada, was bound, gagged, and strangled to death in her own apartment by two brothers who wanted only her bank card. The reality is that a woman doctor in Florida was abducted from her office, forced to hand over her bank card, and then brutally stabbed to death.

Step two in any effective security program is to insist on your right to be protected. It is the responsibility of banks (or any other business) to anticipate dangers and provide consumers with adequate physical security.

Step three in any effective security program is to learn about criminal tactics and to recognize your own responsibility for personal security.

REDUCING THE RISK

1. Use only well-lighted ATMs that are in public view and park your car in a well-lighted area.

2. Avoid ATMs with nearby bushes and other obvious hiding places.

3. Avoid ATMs that offer an easy escape route for a criminal. Think like a criminal! If you were a criminal, could you steal money without being seen or interrupted and then escape from view within seconds? If the answer is yes, you should use a safer ATM.

4. Have someone accompany you while making a deposit or withdrawal. Although this will not always prevent you from becoming a victim, it will reduce the chances of a robbery. If the ATM

is on a street corner or other wide-open area, your "lookout" can watch from inside a locked car. If you don't have a car, the lookout should position herself/himself ten to fifteen feet away. There are scores of cases in which couples standing side by side have been robbed. The purpose of the lookout is primarily to be a visible deterrent. A lone gunman can't easily control both of you so he chooses another target. A visible lookout makes a criminal nervous.

5. Do not make deposits at the same time or place every day. Criminals watch for routine deposits. Warning: If you are in the habit of making large deposits or withdrawals, the chances are good that the word will get out.

6. You are safer if the ATM is in a public area with lots of people mingling about. The criminal worries about witnesses, good samaritans getting involved, and armed off-duty police officers.

7. Even though thousands of ATM-related crimes have occurred during the day, you are still safer conducting business in daylight hours. You also reduce the chances that one crime (a robbery) will turn into other crimes, i.e., kidnapping, rape, murder.

8. Conduct an informal security survey of your ATM. The bank is inviting depositors on the premises twenty-four hours a day; they have a responsibility for your security! Is the ATM in plain view of the public? (You want to be seen.) Is the area well lighted? Are security cameras in place? Are there security guards in the area? Are there places a criminal could easily hide? Does

the door lock behind you? Can you park your car close by in a safe, well-lighted area? (Many robbers follow ATM users to their cars.) Ask the bank, "Have any robberies occurred here?" How safe is the area surrounding the ATM? In many cases banks do not evaluate the security of an ATM or its location until *after* someone has been kidnapped, raped, or murdered.

9. Do your business quickly. The less time you spend at the machine, the less chance you'll be targeted.

10. Do not conspicuously count your money at the machine.

11. Even if the ATM is only a few steps away, do not leave your car running or the keys in your car while at the ATM. Many cars are stolen while the owners are outside the vehicle using an ATM. And almost every victim is wide-eyed with shock when they see their car disappearing at a high rate of speed, especially when a child or pet is still in the backseat! Lock your doors!

12. When using a drive-up machine, be sure all windows (except the driver's) are closed and the doors are locked. Keep your engine running. Be observant. Many of the most heinous of ATM crimes (kidnapping, rape, murder) would have been prevented if the victim had locked her door. The author has read thousands of crime reports against motorists that began with, "The criminal grabbed the door handle, opened the unlocked car door, and . . ." Lock your doors!

13. Do not let others see you put your personal iden-tification number (PIN) into the ATM. Do not

give your PIN to anyone, especially a caller. Do not write your PIN on your ATM card.

14. Since hundreds of ATM customers have been surveilled, watch to see if you are being followed. If you think you are being followed, go directly to a police station or drive to a well-lighted public place and phone police. It will be of great assistance to law enforcement if you can provide a description of the car, the driver, and license plate number.

15. Be aware of your surroundings and never approach an ATM if your instincts tell you it is dangerous.

16. Beware of con artists who are using a variety of schemes to obtain your PIN. After stealing purses many criminals will telephone the victim and pretend to be either the police or a bank official. "We think we've caught the man who stole your purse," the impostor says. "We need your PIN to determine if he has stolen any money from your account."

4

Security at Pay Telephones

On November 12, 1992, at 10:40 A.M., a forty-four-year-old woman was driving through a Maryland suburb en route to work when she realized she was going to be late for a meeting. Spotting a telephone, the woman pulled her car into a shopping center parking lot and called her office. "I'll be a bit late," she told her secretary. As she turned to walk toward her car parked five feet away a young man approached and asked for directions. As the woman was explaining that she had never heard of the address in question, the man pulled a knife, held the blade to the woman's ribs, and forced her into her car with him. "Drive where I tell you or I'll cut your throat," he ordered. The woman drove a couple of miles to a secluded part of the town and was viciously raped.

An estimated 27,000 crimes, including murder, rape, kidnapping, car theft, and robbery of purses, briefcases, and wallets occur at pay telephones each year in the United States. These 27,000 crimes occur during the day and night, at pay phones located at shopping centers, train stations, airports, service stations, and street corners in the best and worst of neighborhoods.

In Long Beach, California, a twenty-three-year-old woman was pulled out of a phone booth at one A.M., dragged behind an apartment building, and raped. In Maryland, a thirty-six-year-old woman was at a phone booth when two men stole her purse and her new automobile. In Washington, D.C., a woman was robbed and stabbed to death when she stopped, late at night, to call her child's baby-sitter from a pay telephone.

From the criminal's point of view there are many strategic reasons for targeting a woman using a pay telephone. First, to use a telephone the victim has to be standing or sitting immobile in one place. A stationary target is easier to surveil and hit than a moving target. Second, a woman using a telephone tends to be engrossed in conversation and usually faces the telephone with her back to the criminal. This, of course, is to the criminal's advantage. Third, while talking at a pay telephone the victim's hands are usually occupied holding the receiver, punching in numbers, putting coins in the telephone, or writing notes. The criminal realizes that if a woman's hands are occupied she cannot grab him, protect herself, or hold on to her belongings.

One criminal who robbed more than thirty people at telephone booths explained that once inside the booth "the target is boxed inside with only one route of escape." He also explained that while a telephone booth helps to drown out street noises it also drowns out screams for help. A professional street thug, this repeat offender would stake out telephones at train stations and shopping centers late at night and break the internal booth light so he could operate in complete darkness.

Although crimes at pay phones occur at all hours and in all neighborhoods, almost 80 percent of the abductions and rapes have occurred at night and/or in extremely isolated areas. In twenty-two attempted rapes studied by the author, the would-be victims were able to escape greater harm by screaming, struggling, or fighting back. Most of the attempted rapes, however, occurred in heavily traveled, populated areas, where help was relatively close by.

In one case a twenty-eight-year-old woman was talking to her boyfriend late at night on a pay phone outside a Pizza Hut restaurant, located in a shopping center, directly across the street from a police station. As she talked, a thirty-one-year-old man on a bicycle approached and began making lewd and suggestive comments. Without warning the man punched the woman in the face and dragged her into her car, which was parked nearby. The man was on top of her in the car, trying to yank her pants down when the woman's screams alerted two men who were driving through the shopping center. The rapist fled on his bicycle when the men, both college football players, approached the car.

In dozens of cases women have had their cars stolen while talking on a pay telephone. Typically, the victim pulled up to a telephone booth, left the keys in the ignition, the engine running and the driver-side door open, while she made a quick call. The carjackers, seeing a target of opportunity, simply jump into the vehicles and drive away.

The most common crime against women at pay phones is the theft of purses, briefcases, and jewelry. Hundreds of women have lost valuables while using pay phones in airports, train stations, shopping centers, etc. In one hundred cases selected at random, seventy-three criminals simply snatched the purse, briefcase, or package and ran. (Frequently the caller was preoccupied and didn't even notice the theft occurring.) In the remaining twenty-seven cases the thieves pulled a gun or a knife and either used violence or ordered the women to give up their valuables. Many of the women who resisted either the "snatch and run" or the armed robberies were injured or killed and still lost their valuables.

On February 20, 1992, two women got lost on Long Island, New York, and stopped to make a phone call. As they stood at the phone two men came up behind them and grabbed their purses. The women resisted, there was a short struggle, and one woman was stabbed in the neck, the other was slashed across her chest. The men escaped with the purses.

REDUCING THE RISK

1. Choose pay telephones located in a populated, well-lighted area. A wide variety of crimes including scores of murders have occurred at pay phones.

2. Do not face the phone with your back to the street or lobby. Face the street, sidewalk, or lobby with your back to the telephone. This way you can still talk on the phone but at the same time be aware of your surroundings and be on the lookout for suspicious-looking characters. If you appear to be alert many criminals will look for an easier target.

3. Maintain physical contact with your purse, briefcase, or luggage. If you cannot hold these items in your arms put one foot on your possessions while you speak.

4. Mobile car phones are an excellent idea for security. There is no question that car phones will

prevent thousands of crimes. But remember, if you are going to be talking on a car phone your first responsibility is to pay attention to your driving!

5. Too many people get out of their car at a phone booth and leave the engine running and the key in the ignition while they make a quick call. Hundreds of cars have been stolen from people who make this mistake. When you get out of your car take your keys and lock your door. It can be a long walk home.

6. Many people make the mistake of placing their wallets on the shelf next to the phone in order to extract coins, telephone credit cards, or a telephone number. A visible wallet is a tempting target. Pickpockets, of course, will watch very carefully to see where you place your wallet. (The man who robbed more than thirty people at telephone booths said, "I just loved those people.")

7. If you are forced to use a telephone booth at night, scan the area for places a criminal might be lurking. Remember, the internal light illuminates and puts a spotlight on you in an otherwise dark area. If the light is out, a criminal may have knocked it out for a reason.

8. If you are with a friend scatter your forces. In other words, one person should make the phone call while the other sits in the car or observes from a distance. This way each person can watch out and assist the other and you reduce the chances that both of you will be victimized. Like soldiers on patrol, don't bunch up, spread out.

Remember, in a desperate situation your vehicle is a powerful defensive and offensive weapon.

9. Many pay telephones, even in populated, well-lighted areas, have at least one hiding place, one blind side, nearby. Before using a phone ask yourself, Where could a criminal hide? One woman using a pay phone in broad daylight was pulled into an innocuous-looking van, parked four feet away.

10. Beware of calling-card theft. Today many criminals are lurking around public telephones hoping to steal calling-card numbers by "shoulder surfing," eavesdropping or peeking over a caller's shoulder. Some more sophisticated criminals are even using binoculars, telescopes, and video cameras to view numbers dialed by card holders. Most calling-card thefts, like most crimes, can be prevented: (a) Speak softly into the telephone when giving numbers to long-distance operators. (b) Block the telephone keyboard from view when punching in a number. (c) Don't be conned into giving out your number to callers who claim to be investigators or someone who is verifying your identity. One man who was conned into giving out his number received a thirty-page telephone bill for $30,146.

11. Remember, you are especially vulnerable to distraction while making a phone call following a long flight. If someone engages you in conversation while making a phone call ("Do you have change?") or if two people on either side of you are talking to one another—be suspicious!

12. Don't argue with someone over petty grievances. The argument might be a staged diversion or you

might be dealing with a "crazy." A twenty-seven-year-old man was killed in a Brooklyn subway station when he asked another man, "Can I use that phone?" The gunman hung up the phone he was using, pulled a shotgun, and shot the man at point-blank range.

5

Attacks on Joggers

The crime that occurred April 19, 1989, under a full moon in New York's Central Park shocked the world with its senselessness and thrust the word *wilding* into our vocabulary.

On that mild spring night a pack of teenagers stalked and attacked a twenty-nine-year-old investment banker as she jogged alone past a grove of sycamore trees. For thirty minutes the boys gang-raped the five-foot-five, 100-pound Wellesley College graduate and brutally beat her with a brick, a rock, and a twelve-inch metal pipe. The "mindless marauders," as a judge would later call them, gagged the woman with her bloody shirt, fractured her skull, and left her naked and unconscious in a mud puddle. When found almost three hours later the woman had lost two-thirds of her blood and had a body temperature of only eighty degrees.

Evincing an unspeakable depravity, this horrible crime against a female jogger symbolizes the violence and fear women must live with in our society. But her recovery stands for strength, courage, and survival. Despite months of painful rehabilitation, despite the psychological trauma, despite her lingering disabilities, this gutsy investment banker has not only resumed her job, she has heroically resumed her jogging.

Millions of women of all ages run or walk for exercise and recreation on a regular basis. The vast majority of these women will enjoy these activities for a lifetime without ever suffering a criminal incident. Nevertheless, in the United States alone at least 7,000 crimes ranging from indecent exposure to assault, rape, robbery, and murder are committed against female joggers each year. Sadly, the impersonal computer printout of "women murdered while jogging" is becoming ominously long. Dozens of women have been stabbed, strangled, beaten, or shot to death while jogging.

Scores of additional attacks against female runners have been nonfatal but shockingly senseless and barbaric. Two men attacked a forty-three-year-old woman who had been jogging in a local park in upstate New York. The woman was beaten, raped, and robbed, and received multiple stab wounds. Using her shoelaces the men tied the woman's hands to sticks that were thrust in the ground. Miraculously, the woman managed to pull free and walk more than two miles for help with a knife protruding from her neck. Fortunately, both men were captured and sentenced to long prison terms.

Unfortunately, sending an offender to prison does not always put an end to the problem. After all, hundreds of prisoners escape each year and thousands of others are released only to commit the same crimes once again.

One day after escaping from prison, a twenty-seven-year-old man attacked, robbed, and raped a woman who was jogging with her dog on a hiker-biker trail. Incredibly, the jogger was attacked only a few blocks from where the man raped another woman several years earlier.

On April 26, 1991, in suburban Maryland, a woman was jogging along a path around a lake when she was dragged into the woods and raped. A teenage boy who was undergoing court-ordered therapy for two previous sexual assaults was charged with the crime. The boy was on a chaperoned field trip with a state juvenile offenders group when he wandered away from his counselors and attacked the jogger.

Many criminals actually specialize in attacking female joggers.

A serial rapist also focused his attention on female joggers. The "South Hill Rapist," as he was called, allegedly raped and beat dozens of women in the Spokane, Washington, area before being caught. Typically, he wore a running suit and jogged the streets in search of female targets. Most of his many victims were either female joggers or women he had followed from a bus stop. On April 24, 1992, a woman was raped while jogging within the confines of her upscale apartment complex in Virginia. A man ran up to her, politely asked if she'd like a jogging partner and she responded, "No, thank you." A few minutes later the same man grabbed the woman, dragged her to a nearby fence (just yards away from heavy pedestrian and vehicle traffic), yanked her pants down, and raped her.

Judging from hundreds of actual incidents, there is no doubt that women are most vulnerable when they are (a) jogging alone, (b) jogging at night, and (c) jogging in isolated, unpopulated areas. However, police files are filled with examples in which female joggers have been victimized in broad daylight in the nicest of neighborhoods. In fact, this data clearly shows that criminals are becoming increasingly brazen and that areas that appear safe are often deceptively dangerous for lone runners. Female joggers, ages thirteen to sixty, have been assaulted in midafternoon while running in the "safest" of neighborhoods and while jogging on high school and college tracks. They have also been attacked while running on golf courses, church property, and populated public parks.

A thirty-seven-year-old was stabbed to death September 19, 1988, as she jogged on a high school track in White Plains, New York. On June 2, 1990, a twenty-two-year-old university student was sexually assaulted and strangled to death while jogging on a bike trail in a bucolic Maryland suburb. When found, she was clad only in a T-shirt and running shoes. Known for its peaceful, small-town atmosphere, this suburb was described by one resident as being "quiet, quiet, quiet." The victim had arrived in Maryland from Houston only three weeks before the attack.

Even in "safe" populated areas, joggers should forego headphones, be aware of their surroundings, and realize that, in this age of violence against women, attacks can occur anywhere.

In scores of reported cases women have struggled free, outrun, or fought off their attackers. A jogger in Boston told the author she escaped a drunk by kneeing him solidly in the groin; in Florida a sixteen-year-old stabbed a long thumbnail into her attacker's eye and he staggered away screaming. Another jogger, grabbed from the front in a bear hug, bit the tip of her attacker's nose off, a tactic that was of great benefit when it came to identifying the perpetrator. "My arms were pinned and I was so scared I just went animal," she said. When asked how they would have responded if their attackers had been armed all three women answered similarly, "I really don't know."

Many other escape tactics have been less dramatic

but equally effective. Screaming is a tactic that has saved many joggers. A woman reported that she was running on a well-traveled path in Alexandria, Virginia, one bright January morning when she noticed a man in street clothes but did not think much about it. Suddenly, the man grabbed her, pinned her arms, and yanked her toward him. Quoted in a newspaper article, the woman said her first reaction was to scream. "I'd never heard such a noise come out of me in my life," she said. "It didn't sound human." The scream startled her attacker and she wiggled free and ran, sobbing and in shock, to safety. The woman was quick to point out that runners aren't just attacked at night. "My attack happened in the daylight."

Shirley Pate, in charge of safety for the Washington RunHers, stated in the *Washington Post* that she was once grabbed while running and has been confronted by exhibitionists on three occasions. Pate says that women should be creative and should not be afraid of looking foolish. "You want to scare your potential attacker and draw attention to yourself."

Sensing she was being surveilled, a jogger in Colorado was certainly being creative when she stared past a stalker, waved to an imaginary friend, and hollered, "Hurry up, Harry!" The would-be attacker turned abruptly and disappeared.

After being dragged into a car and gang-raped by four men in broad daylight, avid runner Shelley Reecher sublimated her rage and fear into a program now called Project Safe Run. A security program with teeth, Project Safe Run in Seattle, Washington, trains "defensive dogs" and rents these dogs to women joggers.

Although traumatized by her ordeal, Reecher refused to stop running but realized she would have to do something about her personal security. She told the author that she tried running with friends but soon learned they were not always available at the times she wanted to run. Then she met Jake, a Doberman pinscher, whom she trained as a "defensive" dog and running partner. A defensive dog is not considered an attack dog but is trained to match an assailant's aggression by barking, growling, and baring his teeth. He or she will only bite if ordered to do so.

Naturally, Reecher's friends also wanted to run with Jake. But since Jake didn't have the time or energy to escort everyone, Reecher eventually acquired twelve more Dobermans, who moved into her one-bedroom apartment.

Affectionately nicknamed "Doberwoman" by her friends, Reecher, quoted in the *Seattle Times,* stated, "Women I didn't even know were calling me and saying they heard that I had these dogs available to run with." She said, "It was amazing how many people this was helping."

Terri Ellis, a client of Project Safe Run, says that Rosie, a pit bull, is a perfect companion. Also quoted in the *Seattle Times* article by Kay Susumoto, Ellis reported that running with Rosie "was a great way to have more freedom and flexibility with my time. With Rosie," she said, "I could be running in the dark and not feel threatened. She gave me a sense of security."

Reecher explained that the size and the reputation of certain dog breeds act as a visual deterrent to crime. Breeds most commonly used by Project Safe Run are Dobermans, rottweilers, German shepherds, Great Danes, and pit bulls.

Project Safe Run currently boasts a perfect record, no accidental bites and no attempted assaults in nearly 12,300 runs.*

Furious that fear should control their lives, women

---

*For more information write Shelley Reecher, 5240 University Way, Northeast, Suite D, Seattle, Washington 98105.

worldwide are facing up to the dangers of jogging but refusing to give up the sport they love. "We don't need to become the scared, shivering gender," stated a woman jogger. "We need to be free. But we also need to be sensible, cautious, and careful."

REDUCING THE RISK

1. Do not stop jogging!

2. The data clearly illustrates that a runner dramatically increases the threat of attack if she jogs alone, jogs at night, or jogs in isolated, unpopulated areas. If possible, try to run with a partner during daylight hours. If you must run alone and/or at night select a well-lighted route with plenty of pedestrian traffic.

3. Many criminal predators stalk their prey and methodically plan their attacks. Don't get into a routine that is easy to monitor. Change your running route frequently and vary the time of day you run. If you must run at the same time each day, e.g., before going to work, consider leaving your house or apartment complex through the front door on some days and the back door on other days. You are noticed by a lot more people than you realize!

4. Remember, many burglars monitor joggers' departures so they can enter an empty house; rapists will enter a home and wait for the jogger to return. Lock your doors! Do not hide your key under the door mat or any other obvious location. In this age of violence you are either poorly informed or denying reality if you rationalize, I'll only be gone for a short while so I'll leave the

door unlocked. It is no exaggeration to say that millions of women have been victimized simply because a door was unlocked.

5. Steer clear of bushes, alleys, dumpsters, parked vehicles, etc., where an assailant could easily hide, reach out, and grab you. Keep in mind that joggers and criminals both enjoy paths through the woods for the same reason: the paths are secluded.

6. If you sense or hear a vehicle slowly approaching, increase the distance between you and the street. If a motorist pulls alongside you and acts in a threatening manner do an abrupt about-face and run in the opposite direction. No matter what the motorist's intentions (to harass, shoot, abduct, hit-and-run), you almost always have a tactical advantage if you run in the opposite direction the car is pointed and then head for a populated area. Be especially suspicious of vans. Always try to get a description of the driver, car, and license plate; this information will probably be saving another child or woman. Do not get paranoid but remember that hundreds of criminals have set up their victims simply by asking directions or asking "Do you have the time?"

7. Criminals don't like to draw attention to themselves. Consider carrying an airhorn or one of several types of battery-operated, ear-piercing personal protection alarms. Many of these noisemakers are quite portable and emit a deafening sound. The advantage of these devices over a whistle is that they can be activated quickly with one hand; many victims have complained, "I never had a chance to put the whistle to my

mouth." If you are struggling with someone or running for your life, it is extremely difficult to continuously blow on a whistle. In addition, there's a good chance you'll lose your teeth if an attacker tries to silence the whistle.

8. Report all cases of indecent exposure and other disturbing incidents. Even though such reports can help police solve past assaults and prevent future attacks, hundreds of "indecent exposure" incidents go unreported. Do not let anyone tell you that male exhibitionists are harmless. On the contrary, scores of rapists, child molesters, and even serial murderers have histories of exposing themselves and masturbating in public. Get angry, get involved, get even; report these incidents to the police!

9. Running or power-walking with a dog—especially a trained Doberman, German shepherd, rottweiler, or pit bull—is an excellent security precaution. There is no doubt that many would-be attackers have changed their mind when confronted with a dog. But don't be lulled into a false sense of security. Even with a trained attack dog you should avoid dangerous areas. Remember, not all dogs will fight for you; some will run off and others will merely watch the assault. In a few isolated cases, determined attackers have shot and killed dogs. Lastly, show some consideration for your dog. Unlike humans, most dogs cannot run long distances at a fast pace without stopping, especially in hot weather.

10. Do not wear headphones. It is a great sacrifice to give these up but it's important for survival. Many women, hearing an attacker close by, were

able to run away or at least avoid being grabbed by surprise from behind. With earphones you cannot hear if someone is shouting a warning; you cannot hear if someone else is screaming for help; you cannot hear the vehicle skidding toward you. Reality dictates that we do not run in a daze. We must stay alert and be aware of our surroundings. A criminal sees headphones on a woman's head and he thinks, Easy target!

11. Use discretion when acknowledging or approaching strangers. Be friendly, but keep your distance and keep moving. When one person distracts you (asking the time, asking for directions, etc.) be aware of what's behind you. If you choose to respond to questions do so on the run.

12. Follow your intuitions and gut feelings; our instincts have served us well since the beginning of time. If something seems "not right" don't question your instincts, just get out of there!

13. Be aware of "jogger robbers" and "runner rapists." As jogging becomes more popular the world is experiencing hundreds of cases in which robbers, rapists, and even political assassins are posing as joggers. During April 1992 police in Houston, Texas, arrested a man charged with twenty-five rapes, burglaries, and assaults. The man chose his targets by jogging through neighborhoods and apartment complexes and looking for open garages, unlocked doors, and female targets. In Washington, D.C., and other cities "jogger robbers" are donning running apparel and robbing people on the street.

14. Carry identification and money for a phone call. Some joggers even carry portable, mobile

phones. The reality, however, is that in 99 percent of all attacks you will not have the luxury or the time to call police, describe your situation and location, and casually wait for the officers to find and rescue you. Nevertheless, if you are unconscious, identification is important. If you are injured, a telephone call can bring assistance and speed up the search for your assailant.

15. Predators seek easy prey. Project self-confidence. The park or path is yours so run like you own it. Do not appear hesitant or fearful. Your body language should project strength. You are a female grizzly bear ready to protect your young. Confidence alone will not assure your safety but in a marginal situation—where the attacker himself is hesitant—looking strong and confident can tip the balance in your favor. Be careful, however, not to become arrogant or to develop an unrealistic sense of invulnerability. Feeling strong and confident does not mean you should run down dark, deserted alleys at night.

6

Hotel Security

Thousands of serious crimes, including rape, robbery, and murder, are committed against women in hotels every year in the United States.

A bank executive was stabbed to death in a nineteenth-floor stairwell of a luxury New York hotel two hours after checking in. She was found with her room key clutched in her hand. In Michigan, a flight attendant was found bound, gagged, and raped with her throat cut at an airport hotel. In Anaheim, California, a teenager was asleep in her hotel room following her high school prom, when she was shot in the head and killed.

Crimes against women occur in the worst and the very best of hotels, and celebrities have never been exempt. Shocked out of sleep, Sophia Loren was once yanked out of bed at the Hampshire House Hotel in New York and forced, at gunpoint, to hand over $700,000 worth of uninsured jewelry. Zsa Zsa Gabor, actress and sex symbol, was once robbed of $625,000 worth of jewels in an elevator at the Waldorf-Astoria in New York. On June 12, 1990, Georgette Mosbacher, cosmetics executive and wife of the former secretary of commerce, was robbed at gunpoint as she got off the elevator on the twentieth floor of the exclusive Barbizon Hotel in New York. The gunman tried to get Mrs. Mosbacher to go into her room with him but she refused and filled his hands with her purse and jewelry worth $40,000. When a nearby elevator opened, Mosbacher dived in, screamed, and sounded the emergency buzzer all the way to the lobby.

Hundreds of women have been raped in U.S. hotels. In 1988, a professional photographer was repeatedly raped by two ex-convicts while she was a guest at a motel in Texas. The photographer's negligence suit was settled for $10 million. Nevertheless, since that incident, three more women have been raped at the same hotel.

Although hundreds of women have been raped in hotel rooms they thought were safe, the 1974 attack on singer Connie Francis in a Howard Johnson Hotel on Long Island is perhaps the most widely known. Francis had returned to her second-floor room about two-thirty A.M. following a performance and was awakened at four A.M. by a knife-wielding attacker. After being viciously raped, the assailant tied Francis to a chair, knocked the chair over, covered her with a mattress, and stole jewelry and a mink coat.

Many criminals, we have discovered, actually specialize in hotel operations. In 1980, a computer programmer for an insurance company killed and mutilated three women in New York hotels. In 1991, a man was arrested for slashing the throat of a woman in a California hotel; he also killed a woman in a Seattle, Washington, hotel. And, unfortunately, the list goes on and on.

The criminals who operate in hotels have dressed and acted like hotel waiters, security guards, chauffeurs, business executives, and aristocrats. Some have been monstrously brutal and others, like the "Gentleman Bandit" (who robbed nearly 100 guests), have been polite and polished.

As might be expected, hotel rapists and robbers use a wide variety of tactics to gain entry to rooms. At a hotel in Maryland, a woman was robbed by a man who posed as a room-service waiter. At another hotel in Maryland, a man posed as a security guard and raped a teenage girl after telling her he had to search her room for drugs. The man who murdered a twenty-year-old in a Houston motel gained entrance to her room by pretending to be with the motel's management.

Many rapists and robbers rely on the "push in" method of gaining entry. After spending the day at Walt Disney World Epcot Center, two women, both in their forties, drove to a motel in Orlando, Florida. As the women were opening the door to their room at about eleven P.M., two men attacked from behind and pushed them inside. Both of the women were robbed and one was raped. To this day the rape victim has difficulty falling asleep, is scared to leave her house, finds that she startles easily, and has had troubles at work.

Scores of criminals enter hotel rooms the easy way; they obtain a passkey and just walk in. A thirty-nine-year-old woman in Florida was in bed in her room at a motel when she heard someone put a key in her door. Suddenly, two men charged into her room, hit her in the head, and tried to put a pillow over her face. The men grabbed her purse, containing $1,000, and her camcorder, and fled.

And then, of course, what easier way to get a key than to own or work at the hotel! A hotel owner was convicted of raping a young woman in his hotel in Indiana. The author receives scores of reports each year in which hotel employees commit crimes in hotels.

The idea that a hotel employee might be a serial murderer or rapist is a chilling thought, especially since there is some precedence. In the mid-1970s a hotel porter in New York killed eleven female guests before being caught. Naturally, he was described as a "quiet, nice man who never got into any trouble."

During one murder trial in Illinois the court found it necessary to sequester the jury in a local hotel. Overnight, four of the jurors' rooms were burglarized as they slept, by someone who had a passkey.

Sometimes the criminal checks into your hotel room before you do, and waits. Every woman's worst nightmare occurred in reality October 31, 1992, when a twenty-year-old woman was raped at a hotel in Orlando, Florida. After she put her sleeping baby daughter on the bed in her hotel room, a man, who had been hiding, jumped the young mother from behind and raped her. The attack occurred shortly after the woman, visiting from the Northeast, was dropped off at the hotel at about eight-thirty P.M. The woman had a difficult time describing her assailant because the lights had just been turned off.

For three years, a Canadian couple planned a dream Christmas vacation to south Florida. But it was the worst Christmas this French Canadian couple had ever experienced. At four-thirty on Christmas morning, two men and a woman burst into their motel room, beat and choked the couple, and robbed them of their car and all of their vacation money. One day in Florida and all they wanted to do was go home, which is no easy task with no car or money.

In a state like Florida, which attracts so many tourists, there are hundreds of hotel horror stories and many of the victims will remember these stories forever. It is unlikely, for example, that a Saudi princess will ever forget the group of pickpockets who stole her briefcase in a hotel near Walt Disney World. The briefcase contained $500,000 in cash and $300,000 in unsigned traveler's checks.

As a microcosm of greater society, anything that occurs in the community, no matter how violent or how bizarre, also occurs in hotels.

Although she had broken up with her jealous boyfriend six months earlier, a Florida woman complained that he continued to follow, harass, and stalk her. Now dating a new man, the woman and her new boyfriend decided to spend Saturday night together in a Florida motel. But the former beau followed them. While the woman was in bed with her new friend the jealous stalker broke into the room and slashed them both with a steak knife. Beating and slashing, the attacker, in a fit of cruel, jealous rage, jumped on top of his rival and mutilated him. As the woman went screaming to the room next door for help, the attacker escaped through a back window. The horribly wounded man was rushed to the hospital. In a state known for hotel horror stories this was one of the most memorable.

While thousands of crimes are committed against women in hotels each year, not all the women are guests; the victim is frequently a hotel employee.

A woman who worked in a Chicago high-rise hotel was raped in a hotel elevator. After holding the elevator door open for a "guest" the woman noticed that the first thing her attacker did was push several floor buttons. Then, as he stood across from her he pulled a handgun and stopped the elevator between floors. The attacker blindfolded the employee with her own scarf, stole her valuables, and then raped her in the elevator.

Scores of women working in hotels, from housekeepers to executives, have been raped, robbed, wounded, or murdered by a wide variety of criminals. In Indiana, an armed robber killed two female front desk clerks at different hotels.

Female housekeepers at hotels tend to be especially vulnerable and often poorly protected. Tragically, several hotel maids, some quite elderly, have been murdered while working alone in isolated rooms. One elderly maid was murdered at a mid-town hotel in New York. She was found in the bathtub, her legs and wrists tied, her body beaten, her throat cut. One week later, in Atlantic City, New Jersey, another elderly maid was murdered. The housekeeper was shot in the forehead and found bleeding between two beds.

In addition to rapes, robberies, and murders, several female guests in 1992 identified a new hotel security problem, one that is making a lot of women nervous. The new problem is *peepholes!* Several lawsuits have been aimed at hotel chains because women have discovered that employees, and who knows who else, have been watching women and men undress, make love, and use the bathroom in hotel rooms. A mother and daughter discovered peepholes in their hotel room in Tennessee. Their attorney has stated, "The only reason for the peephole being there is for employees of the hotel to watch people undressing, showering, or involved in sexual intercourse."

In February 1992 a South Carolina jury awarded $10 million to five hotel guests because of peephole complaints. A judge reduced the amount to $500,000.

A banking executive in New York told the author she had a shocking peephole experience while staying in a hotel in the Middle East several years ago. Thinking that the bathroom mirror over the sink might be concealing a medicine cabinet, a place to store some cosmetics, she gave the mirror a tug. To her horror the mirror fell from the frame, revealing a man staring straight at her from an adjoining room. The mirror was a one-way glass that allowed a viewer to see the entire bathroom and the bed if the bathroom door was left open.

Crime against female guests and employees in the hotel environment is a growing problem that has yet to be properly addressed. Incredibly, many hotels still ignore some of the most basic security precautions.

REDUCING THE RISK

1. Realize that thousands of robberies, rapes, murders, and other crimes occur against women in hotels each year. Even if a hotel has excellent security, every individual is ultimately responsible for her own protection. Use all locks.

2. Even if your room is on a top floor, criminals can jump from one balcony to another. Make sure your balcony doors are locked.

3. Do not open your door until you are satisfied that the caller has a legitimate purpose. Don't be afraid to call the manager or the front desk if you question someone's authenticity. When room service arrives, many women insist that the waiter slip the receipt under the door. It's unlikely an impostor will have a receipt, just a uniform.

4. Be suspicious of any caller who requests to enter your room to check the smoke alarm, the message light on your phone, the television, etc. Verify such requests with the front desk.

5. If someone knocks on your door and then claims to have the wrong room when you respond, report the incident to security.

6. Don't let the bellhop yell out your name or room number when he/she escorts you to your room.

7. Have the bellhop check out your room (closets, shower, under bed, behind curtains) before departing.

8. Dozens of "push in" incidents have occurred when a woman put her key in the door and a criminal shoved her inside. Be aware of men and women loitering about. Ask for escorts to your room.

9. Remember, criminals have frequently pretended to be hotel managers, waiters, security guards, and maintenance personnel. In Houston, Texas, a woman was robbed and murdered in her hotel room by a man who pretended to be the hotel manager.

10. When you leave your room put the Do Not Disturb sign on the door to give the impression that your room is occupied. (Call the maid when you are ready to have the room cleaned.) Many people also leave the television on when they depart the room.

11. Do not use your name when answering the phone; just say hello.

12. When inside the room, secure all locks. If your room has a door to an adjoining room be sure that door is secured also. Many travelers place a chair or other object near the front door. If someone opens your door while you are in the shower or asleep it will hit the chair and make a noise. The noise may discourage or slow the

criminal and it will alert you. Small personal beeper-sized motion alarms are available that will alert you and scare intruders.

13. Be suspicious of telephone callers who ask you to meet them in the lobby or outside. This tactic has been used against hundreds of hotel guests, but mostly outside the United States. One American in a foreign country received a call in his room from a "manager" who asked him to come down to the manager's office because of an emergency. The American was suspicious, called the front desk, and learned that the call was a hoax. The American prevented his own kidnapping. In the Philippines, criminals were luring male and female guests outside hotels by calling rooms and pretending to be with the guest's company. After dozens of guests were robbed some hotels were obliged to post warnings about this tactic.

14. Many people have access to your room. Do not leave valuables, airline ticket information, or business documents where they can be stolen or viewed.

15. Be very careful about who you invite to your room. Hundreds of hotel guests, male and female, have been drugged and robbed.

16. Do not offer too much information about yourself to taxi drivers, bellhops, or maids. These people are occasionally members of criminal networks. Scores of crimes against hotel guests were a direct result of the information the guest gave the taxi driver who brought her/him from the airport.

17. When checking in and checking out of the hotel do not leave your briefcase and luggage out of sight. It's better to escort baggage handlers to and from your room.

18. In case of fire or other emergency be sure you know where all exits are located. Think about an escape contingency plan before you need it.

7

Protect Your Keys

You should no longer think of your keys as a hunk of cheap metal. Your keys, made of diamonds and gold, are worth millions of dollars and should be treated as such. Because with your keys a criminal has access to you and all your treasures: your family, friends and co-workers, your home, your office, your company's secrets, your car.

It is estimated that over 300,000 crimes are committed each year in the United States alone by criminals who have surreptitiously obtained keys to private homes, apartments, offices, cars, and so forth.

In an exclusive Maryland suburb, police continue to search for the body of a young college graduate, who disappeared from the bedroom of her family home. Because of blood and other evidence it is now almost certain that she was bludgeoned to death in her own bed and then transported to an unknown location. Her mother has stated, "whoever came in had a key," and since the slaying the family members have made the sickening discovery that two extra house keys are missing. Police arrested a man who had worked as a gardener and handyman for the family and charged him with the murder. The man, who had bathroom privileges and was allowed to wander in and out of the house, is also the prime suspect in the disappearance of a young girl who vanished while playing in the backyard of her father's Maryland home.

Unfortunately, there are thousands of horror stories concerning keys. A nurse left her purse unattended in a vending machine lunchroom at the hospital where she works. A drug addict stole the purse and, using the keys and information inside, burglarized the nurse's home and murdered her two children. In New York, a gang of street thugs robbed and killed an executive in his limousine. With the victim's keys and wallet, the thugs hopped on a subway and went to the executive's home, where they raped, robbed, and tortured his wife and daughter. In Maryland, a forty-two-year-old woman was abducted from her car, strangled, and shot to death while driving home from work. Police later discovered that the purpose of the slaying was to obtain the victim's house keys in order to abduct her twenty-two-year-old daughter. Using the keys, the daughter was kidnapped and held captive in a motel before escaping.

In thousands of reported cases muggers and purse snatchers have stolen keys and then used those keys to burglarize homes and offices. Scores of these burglaries led to rapes and murders of residents and workers.

Just before Christmas, in a pleasant section of Washington, D.C., a seventeen-year-old woman who lives with her parents was robbed of her purse at knife point in the hallway of her apartment building. The next day the mugger, using the stolen keys, entered the family's apartment and stole cash and Christmas gifts.

When your keys are stolen notify the other people

in your home or office and have your locks changed immediately.

If you wouldn't leave a million in cash sitting on the front seat of your parked car, then you shouldn't leave your purse and keys on the front seat of your car. If a criminal steals these keys it may be eight hours before you even realize the keys are missing; a rapist or a robber can do a lot of damage in your home during that eight hours. In fact, as in many cases, he may be inside waiting for your arrival.

In Maryland a man stole a woman's purse from her car, broke into her apartment with the stolen keys, and located the woman's ATM number in a pile of personal papers. Using the secret password, he cleaned out the woman's bank account. In an almost identical case another man stole a briefcase from a woman's car, broke into her home, and raped her sleeping thirteen-year-old daughter.

It is important to brief your children about key security; explain the cause and effect of carelessness and tell them to notify you immediately if the keys are stolen or lost.

A chain of events in Baltimore led to the death of a family member. Wanting to rob a house, three men abducted a young boy on the way to school and stole his keys. The gang later used the keys to enter the boy's home, where they shot the boy's older brother, who had responded to the noise.

Similar incidents involving keys and children have been reported in almost every state. In Illinois two youths stole keys from student lockers at a local high school. The youths used those keys to burglarize several homes.

Incredibly, thousands of people provide an extra set of keys to workmen, real estate agents, renters, guests, etc., without ever considering the possible consequences. In Wichita, Kansas, a thirty-seven-year-old man and his two daughters, ages nine and sixteen were murdered in their own home by a man who also stole the family car and other valuables. The three bodies were discovered by the man's wife when she returned home after visiting relatives. The murderer, who was later captured, had been a workman in the victims' home and had been given keys so he could install a solarium while the family was away.

Many people, forgetting that keys can be easily duplicated, have a false sense of security when loaned sets of keys are returned. The harsh reality, however, is that if someone duplicated those keys (it's done all the time!) the duplicates can be used that night or a year later. True, most people are honest and law abiding. But even keys loaned to an honest, trusted person are a risk to your security if that person knows dishonest people; if that person is careless about security. In scores of cases, sets of keys given to trusted housekeepers, chauffeurs, baby-sitters, and so forth have been stolen or duplicated by one of their friends or family members.

There are many cases in which keys are stolen from trusted friends, employees, and even family members and then used in a criminal enterprise. In February 1992, police in Orlando, Florida, finally captured a man who burglarized a school on several occasions. The burglar was the twenty-year-old son of the school's caretaker. He had stolen the passkey from his father.

Passkeys, of course, present a huge problem for apartment buildings, dormitories, hotels, and office buildings. If someone steals the passkey he or she has access to every apartment, every room. Management naturally will assure you that access to passkeys is "tightly controlled." Don't count on it! Security for passkeys is notoriously lax. In fact, numerous rapes and robberies in apartment buildings and hotels were committed by criminals who had a passkey.

Ominously, many managers who claim to have a tight control on passkeys don't have the vaguest idea of what security entails. One rape victim discovered that the passkey to her apartment complex had been signed out to 112 people in one year, including outside painters, plumbers, potential tenants, and a slew of security guards who had never undergone a background investigation. Since these people were not escorted, there was nothing stopping them from entering apartments or making a duplicate key for themselves. Furthermore, four passkeys were reported "lost" (no action taken) and nighttime front desk clerks had unsupervised access to the keys. This "tight security" got at least one woman raped.

Women at the University of Florida in Gainesville were naturally upset to learn that over the weekend of January 17–19, 1992, a burglar broke into a campus office and stole two master keys that opened the exterior doors to the dormitories and the rooms belonging to the students. The women had a right to be upset; five University of Florida students were murdered and mutilated by a serial murderer in 1990. By the way, not only was it relatively easy for the burglar to steal these keys—keys that offered access to about 2,200 students in nine dormitories—but the keys were kept in an unlocked desk drawer and the theft was not discovered for a few days.

It's also kind of scary to learn, as we often do, that locksmiths have been convicted of committing crimes in homes and buildings where they installed the locks or made keys. In Cook County, Illinois, for example, a hardware-store employee was convicted of fatally stabbing a woman after he entered her apartment with a key he copied.

Protect your keys, they provide access to you, your loved ones, and your most valuable treasures.

REDUCING THE RISK

1. Understand that a wide variety of criminals want your keys and they will utilize many different tactics to obtain them. Think, what could a criminal do if he/she had my keys? Do not treat keys like a cheap hunk of metal; they are worth millions of dollars.

2. When you move into a new house, fire a housekeeper, lose a tenant, or lose your keys, change your locks. One single mother with three children moved into a new house but did not change the locks. When they were burglarized six weeks later the author discovered that the former owners had given sets of keys to sixteen workmen, real estate agents, and college students who had rented the home as a "group house."

3. If your keys are stolen, notify the other occupants of your home and change your locks immediately.

4. Don't be so trusting! You can't give a set of keys to every workman, realtor, and guest that comes to your home.

5. If you have two locks on a door, have one locksmith change the top lock and a second locksmith change the bottom lock. This will help protect against dishonest locksmiths.

6. If you *must* leave your key in the ignition at a parking lot, do not leave your trunk key or your house keys on the same key ring.

7. One woman took her station wagon to a local mechanic and requested a tune-up, "Because we're driving to California for two weeks." She left her house keys with the ignition key while she did some shopping. When she and her family returned from California the house had been "picked clean" by burglars. Don't leave your key in the ignition, don't announce that your home will be empty for two weeks.

8. When you have keys duplicated at a hardware store, do not leave your name and address, do not pay with a check or credit card that identifies your address. Pay cash, don't give your name.

9. A young woman subleased an apartment in Houston during August 1992 in order to work at the Republican convention. The man who rented her the apartment returned with his own key and bludgeoned her to death. When subleasing an apartment, even for a short while, insist that the locks be changed.

10. In case of carjacking do not keep your car keys and your house keys together on the same key ring. You don't want to lose your car *and* your house. Besides, after losing your car you sure don't want to be locked out of your house!

11. Do not put your name and address on your keys. (If you don't know the reason for this policy, perhaps you should read this chapter over again!)

12. When you are staying in a hotel, hide your home and office keys. Yes, unfortunately it's true. Sometimes criminals have your keys mailed to

an accomplice in your hometown. (They get your address off your luggage or from the front desk, etc.)

13. Don't leave keys out when you are having a party or open house. Would you leave $20,000 in cash laying out if you had a party? Your keys are worth much more!

14. Don't leave your hotel key on your towel while you go in for a swim.

15. Remember, one security mistake (for example, leaving your purse and keys on the front seat of your car) can lead to many crimes.

16. Explain to children that they should notify you immediately if their keys are lost or stolen.

17. There's no harm in giving keys to an honest, trusted friend. But you must ask yourself, Is this person naive or careless about security? Does this person have dishonest friends? Does this person understand the power of these keys?

18. Insist that management protect you. Quiz them about passkeys. Demand that they be responsible. If they do not practice responsible security, if they "just don't get it," then do something for women everywhere—sue their pants off! Policy will change for the better.

19. Hundreds of criminals have used an age-old trick to gain entry to apartment complexes and other locked installations. Carrying groceries or other articles, they stand at the door or gate and pretend to be fumbling for their keys. You, seeing

the struggle, open the door with your key and politely let them in. Don't fall for this trick. You may be helping someone commit a serious crime. Don't be an unwitting accomplice. If they don't have their own key don't let them in.

8

The Impersonation of Police (or Phony Police)

An astonishing 25,000 women, men, and children are victimized by police impersonators every year in the United States. Criminals posing as police have stopped, robbed, and raped female drivers; invaded private homes; kidnapped executives; molested children; and conned widows out of life savings. The impersonation of police is one of the most common and certainly one of the scariest criminal tactics in use today.

A particularly unsettling aspect of the police impersonation phenomenon is that it's a tactic so commonly used by serial murderers and rapists. In fact, scores of serial murderers and sex offenders worldwide have incorporated the police impersonation tactic into their psychotic repertoire, and women are most frequently the victims.

Ted Bundy killed numerous women in the United States. Although he used a variety of ruses and props to win the confidence of his victims, he was known to have flashed a badge and stated, in effect, "I'm a police officer, miss, would you come outside with me—your car has been broken into."

Two men dubbed the "Hillside Stranglers" in California tortured, raped, and strangled at least ten women ages twelve to twenty-eight. Their favored tactic was to pose as California Highway Patrol officers. The demented duo would stop a female motorist or pedestrian, show her a police badge, and state, "Police officers, ma'am, may we see some identification?" After accusing the innocent victim of some trumped-up crime, the two impostors would order, "You'll have to come with us." The poor victim would be handcuffed, stuffed into the back of an unmarked car, and never seen alive again. On one occasion it's believed that the Hillside Stranglers kidnapped, raped, and strangled two women simultaneously. As the women were strolling down the street the two men reportedly drove up, produced police badges, and warned the women that an armed psychopath was loose in the neighborhood. The young women were told it would be safer to ride with the "police."

Police impersonators are committing crimes against women in all fifty states, crimes that increasingly include rape.

In Washington, D.C., a thirty-two-year-old woman reported that she was driving home after dark when a car with a flashing light on the dashboard pulled her over in a secluded area. A man in civilian clothes who said he was a policeman told the woman she was suspected of drunken driving. Although the woman had not been drinking, she presented her driver's license as ordered and stepped out of the car. At that point the impostor grabbed the woman by the neck, dragged her into the woods, and raped her.

During 1992 a woman was raped every week on the nation's highways, frequently by police impersonators. In Philadelphia a man pretending to be a plainclothes police officer entered the passenger side of a woman's vehicle, pointed a handgun, and ordered her to drive to a secluded area, where she was raped. At eight P.M., a woman was pulled over on the New Jersey Turnpike by a man with a flashing blue light on his dashboard. After displaying a badge, the man pulled a gun and forced the woman to perform a sexual act in the backseat of her car. At one A.M., in Maryland, a man turned on a flashing light in a car that resembled an unmarked police car and pulled a woman to the side of the road. The man ordered the woman out of the car, forced her to the side of the road, and sexually assaulted her.

So what's the good news? The good news is that in over 100 cases reported to the author, female motorists and pedestrians have *thwarted* attacks by police impersonators.

In Georgia, a woman pulled over by a car with flashing red lights took one look at the battered police car and the shabbily dressed man walking toward her and put her foot to the floor. But the man put on his flashing lights again and chased the woman at speeds hitting ninety miles per hour. At one point the man pulled in front of the woman trying to force her to stop, but she went around. Six miles down the road the would-be victim spotted a marked police vehicle at a shopping center and told the officer about the chase, as the impostor, with lights still flashing, whizzed by. The officer gave chase and, finally, stopped and arrested the impostor.

But different women have thwarted phony police in different ways. A twenty-one-year-old Pennsylvania woman was frisked indecently by a man in a police-style uniform. Probably thinking, Something is very wrong here!, the woman assertively demanded to see proper identification and the impostor fled.

A police impostor in Virginia was thwarted when a

woman refused to unlock her door and demanded to see identification. The young woman was pulled over for speeding at ten P.M. by a car with flashing lights and several antennas. When the impostor, in his mid-twenties, began shaking her locked door handle, the woman stepped on the gas and drove for help.

In Wisconsin, a woman driving alone was pulled over at eight P.M. The man claimed to be a state patrol officer but the woman's instincts said something was amiss. She kept her doors locked and attempted to contact police with her CB radio. The man fled when he saw the radio.

A number of other women, ordered into unmarked vehicles by police impostors, have been able to push free and flee on foot when the situation became obviously suspicious. A twenty-two-year-old woman, stopped for "suspected drunk driving" in Annapolis, Maryland, was ordered to move over to the passenger side of her vehicle so the "officer" could drive. The phony cop turned into a private driveway, grabbed the woman, and ordered her into the backseat. Fortunately, the woman was able to break free and ran to a nearby house to call police. The impostor escaped with the woman's Jeep.

As might be expected, many police impersonators are serial rapists who attack repeatedly. When police in California finally arrested a man dubbed the "Impostor Rapist" they charged him with an incredible sixty-one counts of rape, assault, robbery, and kidnapping. Reportedly, he drove around town in a car that resembled a police undercover vehicle and would pull up to female pedestrians, quickly flash a badge, and order the women inside his car. But for every woman he victimized another woman escaped harm. Apparently, the women who escaped harm stood a few feet from the car, requested to see photo identification and badge, and in some cases requested that a uniformed officer be sent to the scene. In each of these cases the "Impostor Rapist" simply drove away. It is believed that the women who obediently obeyed the impostor's orders, despite serious suspicions, were driven to secluded areas and attacked.

Women in the United States have frequently been kidnapped—from the street, homes, and hotels—and held for ransom by men and women who posed as police officers.

In one of the most notorious kidnappings in American history, a kidnapper and his accomplice posed as police, broke into a Decatur, Georgia, hotel room, and kidnapped Barbara Jane Mackle on December 17, 1968. Mackle, a twenty-year-old student at Emory University, was buried alive in a coffinlike box in an attempt to extort $500,000 from her father, a wealthy former General Development Corporation official. Heroically, Mackle survived eighty-three hours in her crypt, despite minimal sustenance and difficulty in breathing, until police and FBI agents rescued her.

More recently, an elderly woman was kidnapped from her home in Virginia by a police impersonator and a fifty-seven-year-old homemaker was kidnapped from her residence in Illinois, by a man posing as an FBI agent. Although both women were traumatized by the experience, both were eventually freed from captivity and the ransoms were recovered.

In several instances, criminals pretending to be police officers have knocked at private residences and stated, "I'm here to inspect your smoke alarm." Homeowners who failed to ask to see identification or failed to be suspicious of this very unusual request have frequently been robbed, beaten, and raped. A woman who attended one of the author's security seminars was prepared when a man claiming to be a policeman requested to inspect her smoke alarm. The woman requested to see police identification (which he did not have) and asked for his captain's name, which he could not produce. The woman kept her door locked, the man departed, and the woman called the police, who told her that the impostor had already raped one woman and robbed three others!

In other cases, criminals in civilian clothes have knocked at private homes, flashed a police-type badge, and asked to interview the occupants concerning "an escaped prisoner" or "several burglaries in the neighborhood." Once inside, the fake police have robbed and terrorized the family members.

During February 1992, in California, four men wearing business suits were pretending to be policemen and telling families they had a warrant to search their homes. Once inside the home, the men would pull guns and rob the victims of cash, jewelry, and cars. None of the victims had inspected the "officers'" badges, credentials, or warrants.

In 1987, police officials in Virginia recorded at least eight cases in which a man, pretending to be a police officer, had burglarized homes. The phony police officer, who ironically claimed to be installing burglar alarms, targeted people over sixty-five years old and stole household items, jewelry and cash. In some cases the impostor hit the elderly residents and threw them to the ground.

Hundreds of people have fallen victim to the "bank examiners" scheme. In this scheme a telephone caller contacts a potential victim and claims he is a detective conducting an internal investigation at the victim's bank. "Ma'am, we need your help to catch a dishonest bank employee," says the fake detective. "We think this employee is stealing from customers' accounts," says the phony officer and "We need you to withdraw $2,000 from your account." The fake detective explains that the cash will be returned the next day. Incredibly, hundreds of women and men have withdrawn large sums of money, given it to phony police officers, and lost their savings. Potential victims need to realize that no real police officers or bank employees will ask a customer to assist in an internal theft investigation. Don't be one of the hundreds of people who are victimized by variations of this tactic every year.

Several banks have reported that fake police officers have approached bank customers and offered to carry their deposit or withdrawal money "because we've had so many robberies." To date, most victims of this scam have been elderly women or foreigners unaccustomed to U.S. banking procedures.

The impersonation of police is one of the most versatile of criminal tactics. It is used by every conceivable type of criminal, including rapists, robbers, burglars, serial murderers, con artists, child molesters, and so on. And it is used in every conceivable location: the street, the home, the office.

REDUCING THE RISK

1. Do not become paranoid (most police you encounter will be real!) but realize that 25,000 women, men, and children are fooled by police impersonators every year in the United States.

2. When the situation warrants concern, ask to see the officer's identification. This is especially true if the "officer" is driving an unmarked car and is wearing civilian clothes instead of a uniform. If the individual comments, "I forgot my badge and identification," you are probably dealing with an impostor.

3. Don't just glance at the credentials, look carefully at the badge and identification. Many impostors use badges and identification that are obviously

children's toys. After noticing that many people
never really inspect credentials, the author, in an
experiment, once pasted a picture of Mickey
Mouse on his law enforcement identification.
During investigations the author showed his credentials to several people but nobody noticed his
photo had been replaced by Mickey Mouse. After
telling one ambassador that he should be more
observant and more careful, the ambassador re-
plied, "Oh I noticed the photo, but I think you
look like Mickey Mouse!"

4. Follow your instincts. If your instincts tell you
    that there is something odd, unprofessional, or
    unusual about the situation, your instincts are
    probably correct. After being victimized by the
    police impersonation tactic, many women have
    stated, "I just knew something was wrong."

5. Frequently, police impersonators use the tele-
    phone to lure victims from their homes or busi-
    nesses or to obtain private information. All of
    these cases could be prevented if the victim
    would verify the authenticity of the caller by
    telephoning the local police. Remember, anyone
    can call your office or home and state, "This is
    Detective Smith." Bankers and store owners will
    sometimes get a call from police impostors say-
    ing, "There's been a break-in; can you come
    down to the bank/store and meet with investiga-
    tors?" When the banker or store owner arrives,
    the phony police order her to open the safe.

6. Don't be afraid to ask polite questions. What is
    the name of your supervisor? What is the tele-
    phone number of your precinct? Could you
    please give me additional information concern-

ing your request? Impostors have often departed when confronted by a potential victim who seems savvy, suspicious, and street smart.

7. If you are stopped under suspicious circumstances by an unmarked police car, keep your doors locked, your engine running, and request to see the officer's badge and identification. This is especially true if you are stopped late at night in an isolated area and you know you have not broken any laws. If you don't feel safe in stopping for an unmarked car, slowly proceed to a place of reasonable safety before pulling over. If you have reason to be suspicious of a plainclothes officer you may ask if he will radio for a uniformed officer before exiting your vehicle.

8. If a plainclothes officer walks right up to you in a restaurant or shopping mall and states, "Someone has backed into your car in the parking lot" be very cautious. Ask yourself, how did this man know where to find me, how did he know I'm the owner of that car? A real policeman wouldn't know; an impostor knows because he's been following you.

9. With a minimum of 25,000 police impersonation incidents each year in the United States, there are naturally many different scenarios depending on the type of crime (rape, kidnapping, carjacking, confidence scams, etc.) and the location of the crime (the street, home, office, etc.). Simply being *aware* of the police impersonation tactic will help prevent you from becoming a victim in most cases.

10. Remember, anyone can get a badge, a flashing dashboard light, a uniform, and a false identification. Anyone can say, "I'm a police officer."

9

Phony Photographers and the Modeling Masquerade

Pretending to be a photographer with a modeling agency, a man handed out fake business cards in shopping malls and lured nine women to their deaths in eight weeks. Another phony photographer is currently serving fifteen years in prison. He lured more than a dozen women to his "studio" with promises of a modeling career, and then drugged, raped, and took pornographic pictures of them. Albert DeSalvo, the Boston Strangler, pretended to be a representative for a modeling agency and killed thirteen women within eighteen months.

Posing as professional photographers, casting directors, and modeling agents, scores of serial murderers and sex offenders have, over the years, victimized thousands of women. In fact, somewhere in the United States, at least one woman becomes a victim of this tactic every single day. Falling for this one single tactic, dozens of women have been murdered, hundreds have been raped or sexually abused, many are still missing, and thousands have had close calls.

But not all women targeted by these fiends and frauds become victims. For every victim, at least five other aspiring models listened to their instincts, had the "photographer" checked out and took appropriate security precautions.

Described as tall, quiet, and ambitious, a young New York woman wanted to be an actress, model, and dancer. Her aspirations led to her death. The body of this pretty young lady, clad only in blue socks, was discovered in a green plastic trash bag in the rear of a Manhattan parking lot. She had been shot once in the head at point-blank range.

If someone told her he had connections, that he could introduce her to important people in the world of modeling, the victim would listen. The killer was that someone. He was a fake, of course, but the man posing as a theatrical agent excited her with promises of fame and fortune. In fact, he excited many young ladies with the same line. But this "quiet, timid," Jekyll-and-Hyde-type character was arrested for the murder of the aspiring model.

Claiming to be a professional photographer, another perpetrator convinced a woman to pose for an alleged advertisement. The woman was very excited and probably harbored secret fantasies that this job could make her famous. But her parents, wiser to the ways of the world, decided to ask questions, lots of questions, and they didn't like the answers. They refused to give their daughter permission to pose. She was furious.

But the fake photographer just shrugged his shoulders, picked up his directory, and called another young woman, one of many who had caught his eye.

Don't give her time to think, time to investigate my story, the "photographer" probably thought. He told the woman that he was on an extremely tight deadline, that the job had to be done that evening.

She was close to her father and reportedly shared the details of this assignment with him. Her father didn't like it, said it sounded unprofessional, fishy. "Don't worry, Daddy, he's married," she reportedly stated. It's assumed her father just rolled his eyes back and thought, So what! When the young woman showed up at the apartment (his "studio") the stage was set with cameras, lights, and other props.

The phony photographer took about thirty photographs of the victim, and then strangled her to death. It is also believed that the woman was the second aspiring model this impostor had murdered.

Phony photographers have also attacked children. In Canada, for example, a young girl had been receiving a lot of publicity because of her accomplishments in track and field. She was in the kitchen with her mother when the phone rang. On the other end was a man who claimed to be a photographer with the local newspaper. He said his paper was doing a story on the young track star and that they needed some photographs. Could she come down to the playground field, a few blocks away, he inquired. The mother told her daughter it would be OK but that she was expected back soon for dinner. Tragically, the little girl never returned. The local newspaper, of course, had not sent a photographer; the man was an impostor.

In several cases, criminal charges have been brought against real photographers and real talent agents. In October 1992, California police arrested a talent agent and booked him for several cases of alleged sexual battery and false imprisonment. The charges, by actresses and models, state that the man allegedly assaulted the women during auditions and interviews.

Another dangerous man was picked up by police in Los Angeles. He was posing as a casting director, charging aspiring actresses "management fees," and soliciting sexual favors when the women visited his "office." Twenty-one women got angry, got together, and got even; he went to jail.

REDUCING THE RISK

1. Understand that hundreds of men have posed as professional photographers, modeling agents, and casting directors. This chapter mentions only a few of the grand total. It's a popular tactic.

2. When approached by a photographer or modeling agent, ask lots of questions and be suspicious of evasive answers. Where is your studio? (Check out the address.) What is the phone number? Who are some of your other models? (Call them and ask additional questions.) What is your boss's name? How long have you been located at this address? Request references. Do you live around here? Where? Show me some of your work.

3. Be suspicious of the man who approaches you at a shopping mall with a camera around his neck and wants to sign you up. It's OK to talk with him in a public place if you choose. After all, he could be for real and it might be a great opportunity for you. Nevertheless, be businesslike, not flirtatious, and do not supply him with your last name, address, or phone number. Have him give you *his* address and phone number. You'd be wise not to sign anything on the spur of the moment. Do not follow him outside or to a "private area" for any reason. "My van is in the parking lot; come on out and I'll give you a release form." Don't do it. When you leave, watch to see if the man is following you (a very

bad sign). Do not let him see your car. You may have just stimulated a potential stalker.

4. When you meet with a photographer it's best if you take someone with you.

5. Don't let desperation (being broke!) dictate your decision making. Think security, then money, in that order. Also, try to determine his desperation. Is he too eager? Is he pressuring you to come with him, now?

6. Don't let your guard down just because the "photographer" is accompanied by a woman. Incredible as it may sound, a number of serial murderers and sex offenders have used "girlfriends" or even female hostages to help them lure additional victims. One serial murderer used a female companion to win the confidence of his victims. Do not go outside with this woman, do not get into a car with her.

7. Say "thank you" to a compliment but do not let it spin your head and cloud your judgment. Don't give up your dreams, but don't give up on reality, either. Yes, you are very beautiful, but is this compliment going to cost you? "Thank you" is good, "I'll follow you anywhere" is bad.

8. If you choose to model nude or semi-nude that's your choice and your business. But some extra precautions are in order here. From a legal and a security point of view you are getting into dangerous territory. Get good legal advice. Ten years from now you may not want these photos in circulation and if they are in print you will want to make sure someone else isn't making all

the money! More important, think security. Check the photographer's references very closely. No matter how cool or nonchalant the "artist," there's no reason you should allow yourself to be fondled or groped. If the conversation becomes sexually suggestive or inappropriate, end the session, it's over; no second chances. Take someone with you to these sessions. Even if the photographer claims it's for an upstanding "academic magazine" or an "educational film" do not allow yourself to be bound, handcuffed, or gagged "for effect."

9. If a situation seems odd don't disregard your instincts. A model murderer, also an exhibitionist, would get out of the shower and "accidentally" walk in on models at his studio. "Sorry, I didn't know you were here," he'd explain to the embarrassed models.

10. Do not meet with photographers and modeling agents in private, secluded, out-of-the-way locations. Be very suspicious if he does not want you to call him (no matter what the excuse) and very suspicious if he does not want to meet in an established, occupied office during normal working hours. Take an escort or two if the photographs are to be taken in the woods or other isolated areas. Let someone know who, where, and why you are meeting.

10

Classified Ads

A man dubbed the "Classified Ad Rapist" allegedly murdered nine women and committed fifty-five rapes in Florida. Scanning the newspaper classified ads, he would call numbers under the "for sale" columns and make appointments with housewives to view the merchandise for sale. Typically, he would arrange to meet with these women at their homes during the day, when he hoped they would be alone. Once inside, he would pull a weapon, tie up the victim, rape her, and then rob the house.

More than 500,000 people in the United States know that they have been victimized by a classified ad placed in a newspaper. At least another 200,000 people have been victimized by classified ads, in numerous ways, but they don't know it.

Criminals use the classified ads—help wanted, for sale, lost, obituaries, wedding announcements, personal ads, and other sections—in a wide variety of ways. By searching the wedding and funeral announcements, burglars are able to determine when the involved families will be away from their homes. Many of these victims have no idea that the burglars read their wedding and funeral announcements in the newspaper. Con artists might search the obituaries for recently widowed, elderly women, in hopes of cashing in on their grief and their deceased husband's life insurance policy. Serial murderers and rapists use the for sale and the personal ads as a way to meet their victims.

Some serial murderers and rapists place their own ad ("Women's Golf Clubs for Sale") hoping to lure you to them.

One killer met some of his victims when he responded to their classified ads selling video equipment. In other cases he offered to purchase advertised cars, but the seller would have to deliver the vehicle to his cabin in the woods, where many victims were later found in shallow graves.

A California man was sentenced to prison for raping four women. Although his victims didn't know it at the time, they all had something in common; they all answered ads he had placed for a roommate.

When one "model murderer" was released from prison for the murder of an aspiring actress, he didn't come out rehabilitated but he did come out retrained. He learned a new way to lure the actresses he targeted. He reportedly put an ad in the newspaper that read: "Actresses, ages 17 to 25, are being interviewed for parts in a motion picture: Contact Mr. Williamson."

Thousands of people each year become victims of some version of the help wanted employment ruse.

Ann Rule, a former policewoman, wrote an excellent book, *The Want-Ad Killer,* about a serial murderer. A monster of a man, he brutalized and murdered several women in the United States over a period of twenty-five years. One of his favorite tactics was to put ads in the newspaper offering employment.

"Wanted: Woman to work as cashier at Harvey's Texaco Station." This two-line ad in a newspaper assured him of a steady flow of potential victims. Usually when a young woman would call inquiring about the job, he would suggest they meet at a location other than his gas station.

Nobody knows how many women he killed because some of the women he came in contact with have vanished.

Con artists use the classified ad employment ruse in many different ways. In one case a group of con artists put an ad in a newspaper offering exciting, well-paying, overseas employment. Interested applicants were interviewed at a local hotel and told to bring their passport and resumé. Following a short interview, each applicant was told to leave his or her passport overnight and to return the next day at the same time. "We'll let you know if you are hired, and return your passport tomorrow," said the interviewer. At least forty-two American passports belonging to women and men were stolen in that scam.

During the Gulf War, when many Americans were desperately unemployed, several scam artists made a killing with misleading advertisements that offered high-paying jobs rebuilding Kuwait. Most of the applicants, who were already short on cash, ended up spending hundreds of dollars for services that, in truth, offered no hope for jobs.

Hundreds of women throughout the United States have reported being victimized by a wide variety of travel-ad scams. It seems like every year women report sending in down payments for once-in-a-lifetime dream vacations, only to find that the "travel agent" doesn't exist or the trip is bogus. In March 1992 the FBI arrested a couple in Fairfax, Virginia, who were selling bogus vacation packages. The couple had taken over $60,000 from customers for vacations they never intended to provide.

Every month the author receives reports of women being robbed when they advertised something for sale. One woman got robbed and then got even.

In Texas, a woman ran a newspaper advertisement offering to sell a diamond ring for $5,000. A man calling himself "Mike Simmons" answered the ad.

They decided to meet in the parking lot of a doctor's office where the man claimed to have an emergency appointment. He got into the woman's car and she showed him the ring. He said, "I'll take it," grabbed it from her and ran from the car.

Police reportedly told the frustrated victim there was nothing to do except to check local pawnshops. But the woman had another idea. She asked a friend to place another advertisement to sell an emerald and diamond ring. "Hi, I'm interested in the ring you advertised for sale," said the man who identified himself as "Mike Simmons." A meeting place was agreed to and the police snatched "Simmons" before he could snatch another ring.

In one case an escaped convict was making a living by answering ads from people eager to sell their Rolex watches. Claiming to be a physician, this con artist asked a few women to meet him at a local hospital where he allegedly worked. The woman would show up in the hospital lobby with her watch and the con artist would greet her wearing a white coat. After inspecting the timepiece the con artist would ask the woman if he could show it to a fellow doctor upstairs who owned a Rolex. When the woman agreed, the con artist would disappear.

A hundred criminals might use the classified ads in a hundred different ways. A single mother with a teenage son responded to a personal ad that she now knows was placed by a man not interested in her, but in young boys. After dating for a while, the man told the woman that her son needed some guidance and that he, as a male role model, should spend more time with him. On one outing the man, a former policeman, tied the teenage boy, whipped him thirty-five times with a belt, and sodomized him. The mother later learned that the man was a convicted sexual predator and had served time for raping another young boy.

More than seventy-five people were duped in 1992 by the "lost pet" scam. In each case the criminals responded to ads placed by people who had lost pets. A couple in Virginia received a call from a man who said he'd found their missing dog. Naturally, they were overjoyed. The caller agreed to meet them on a street in Washington, D.C. When they arrived, the man got in their car and he directed them to an apartment where, he said, his sister was keeping the dog. On the way, the man explained there was a small matter of a veterinarian's bill. He also explained that since his sister's children had grown attached to the dog he would like money to buy them a new puppy. After they gave the man cash he went into the apartment to get the dog and never returned.

REDUCING THE RISK

1. If you are selling something at your home, it's best if you are not alone when the buyer arrives to inspect the merchandise.

2. If you are meeting someone who has advertised an item for sale, meet in a public place. Don't go alone and don't hand over cash until you have possession of the purchase.

3. Be advised that several people who advertised cars for sale were robbed of that car when the prospective buyer asked for a test drive.

4. If you are responding to a job offer be suspicious if that person doesn't want to meet on the premises. Do not answer inappropriate questions. Do not give out your address or phone number until you've checked out the offer. One serial murderer asked his applicants questions of a personal and sexual nature. Do you live alone? Will you be taking the bus or hitchhiking to work? Do you have a boyfriend? The women who refused to answer his questions are survivors.

5. If responding to a job ad, ask questions, and obtain information about the company and your contact. Make sure the offer is legitimate. One perpetrator told dozens of women who answered his "actresses wanted" ad that he was a Ph.D candidate, that he was working on an educational film about women, that he owned a production company, and that his name was Williamson. All this information was false and could have been checked out.

6. Be especially cautious when responding to ads for models, actresses, flight attendants, overseas employment, or "Beautiful, sexy girls wanted for . . ." Be cautious of ads asking for women to participate in studies of a questionable nature.

7. Understand that if you put an ad in the paper announcing a wedding or funeral, burglars might find this information titillating. Captured burglars have frequently had piles of obituary and wedding notices in their pockets. Some burglars

scan local papers for names of high school football players. The burglars then look up the player's address, and visit that home while the football games are being played. The burglar figures the player's family will be at the game and the house will be empty.

8. The personal ad, once disdained as the meeting place for the desperate and weird, has vaulted into respectability. Many women who work and commute long hours and shun the bar scene have established meaningful relationships through personal ads. Nevertheless, you still have to be careful. Don't give out too much information at first. Take it slowly. Talk on the phone a few times before going out with your date; your instincts will tell you a great deal. Meet in a safe public place. Take charge of your life, take a chance at meeting a compatible partner, but don't take a chance with your security.

9. Don't stop putting ads in the paper and don't stop responding to ads in the newspaper. But in every situation use some street sense and think security. Think! How might this ad endanger me? Then take precautions that will reduce the risk.

11

Pickpockets and Bag Snatchers

While window shopping at a mall in Maryland, a thirty-seven-year-old nurse was approached by a friendly college-aged couple walking arm in arm. "Did you know you have ketchup on the back of your blouse," asked the cute "coed." "Oh, no!" the nurse screeched. Without hesitation the nice young lady produced a Kleenex and helped the nurse clean the ketchup that someone had squirted over her left shoulder and back. Unfortunately, while the exasperated nurse was being cleaned up by this helpful couple, she was also being cleaned out; the man had stolen her wallet from her purse and dropped it into his shopping bag. The nurse had just joined a list of thousands of people to be victimized by the "ketchup squirt" pickpocketing technique.

The wealthy woman who landed at an international airport in Texas following an exhausting, fourteen-hour overseas flight was tired and jet-lagged and did not notice that three men and a woman were following her through the airport. The woman did not notice the four innocent-looking criminals, but the criminals noticed the woman's expensive jewelry and clothes and her Vuitton luggage. After hailing a taxi, the woman gave her luggage to the driver, put her Vuitton bag in the backseat, and pushed her cart about ten feet back to the sidewalk. As she pushed the cart, she, the taxi driver, and the taxi dispatcher were simultaneously approached by three men with questions. The woman's Vuitton bag was gone when she returned to the taxi. The expensive bag contained her passport, over $4,000 in cash and, incredibly, over $200,000 worth of jewelry!

A thirty-seven-year-old woman, visiting California for the first time on a business trip, was breakfasting alone in the coffee shop of an upscale hotel in downtown Los Angeles. While waiting for her bill to be delivered she was sipping on a cup of coffee and mentally rehearsing a presentation she would be delivering in Hollywood at ten-thirty A.M. As she scribbled a few reminders to herself on a notepad, a well-dressed gentleman in his thirties approached and nonchalantly commented, "Excuse me, but I think you've dropped some money under the table." The woman put down her pen, picked up the edge of the tablecloth, and sure enough a wad of crumpled dollar bills were by her left foot. In the few seconds it took the woman to reach under the table the man had grabbed the woman's briefcase from the chair next to her and disappeared. Actually the thief was so smooth that the woman didn't even notice the briefcase was missing until she got up to leave a couple minutes later. And then panic set in! Her briefcase contained cash, credit cards, some "very personal" letters from her fiancé and important business papers. Without the briefcase there was no reason for the ten-thirty meeting and no reason to be in California. She was devastated.

What the woman didn't realize is that the "crumpled money" tactic has been used hundreds of times.

After the initial shock of losing her briefcase the woman had to deal with reality. Embarrassed, she had to apologize for canceling her meeting ("God, they probably think I'm a dingbat," she told the author); she sheepishly explained to her clients back east that their papers were now in the hands of a stranger. And then, of course, there were other practical matters: "How will I pay for taxis and the hotel?" "My house keys were in the briefcase." "Those letters were very personal."

Like swarms of locusts, pickpockets and bag snatchers swoop down on shopping malls, airports, hotels, train stations, and street corners and victimize over 500,000 people each year in the United States. Like the nurse, the wealthy woman at the airport, and the businesswoman in California, these 500,000 people are victimized because they don't know how criminals operate.

The Ketchup Squirt

The "ketchup squirt" technique is currently being used in over fifty countries and has claimed thousands of victims in the United States alone. It is one of the most popular pickpocketing techniques in use today but, like the nurse at the shopping mall, millions of potential victims have not been warned. Police are reporting this technique being used in airports, shopping malls, train stations, restaurants, and in the street.

Typically, the pickpocket punctures a pinhole in a small package of ketchup usually found in fast food stores. The pickpocket then squeezes the package, forcing a stream of ketchup onto the clothes of his or her victim. One or two members of the pickpocketing team then inform the victim, "Excuse me, miss, did you know you have ketchup on the back of your coat?" While the team members help the victim clean the ketchup they are also stealing a wallet from a pocket or purse. Sometimes the good samaritan offers to hold the woman's purse while she cleans up; sometimes the victim sets her purse and purchases on the ground while she cleans up; and sometimes, in the confusion, she doesn't notice that the purse, hanging over her shoulder, has been opened. Not all pickpockets use ketchup. Some use barbecue sauce, mustard, or any other condiment of their choosing.

One twenty-three-year-old woman who had been briefed on this tactic was able to thwart an obvious pickpocketing attempt at Miami International Airport. "As soon as they told me I had the ketchup on my coat I squeezed my purse tightly, backed away, and took off my coat," she said. "It was really kind of comical how they kept offering to hold my purse," she said, "but I'm still angry they squirted ketchup on my coat."

Escalator Dancing

In a subway station in Washington, D.C., a woman was nearing the top of an escalator when she noticed a well-dressed woman who appeared to have her shoelace caught in the machinery. "I had to do a quick dance to avoid tumbling on top of her," the woman said. People behind the woman were also "dancing" to avoid a pileup. Moments later the victim looked down and noticed that her purse was open. She realized immediately that her wallet had been stolen. Before the woman could cancel her credit cards the thieves had charged almost $3,000 worth of merchandise. As we so often see in the security business, one crime (a stolen wallet) leads to other crimes (use of credit cards). Had the woman lost her house keys they may have been used to burglarize her home.

Thieves on escalators are using a variety of tactics. Sometimes they spill coins on the moving escalator steps and then walk in place, trying to pick up the coins. This causes other riders to step back, falling into the arms of pickpockets. Sometimes one of the accomplices pretends to trip and fall, causing a commotion, a pileup, and easy pickings. Frequently, an escalator thief will steal from a victim going up the escalator and literally pass his loot to an accomplice going down the escalator.

The "escalator dance" has been so successful for the criminals there is no doubt that it will continue to be used.

Elevator Crunch

As people squeezed into the parking-garage elevator at a hotel in Atlantic City, New Jersey, a woman screamed, "Too close! Too close!" while an accomplice reached into a customer's pocket and stole $1,429 in casino winnings. A few minutes later on another elevator the woman again screamed, "Too close! Too close!" and the pickpocket team stole $820. When the pickpocket team was arrested they were found to have three straight razors (for protection and for slashing pockets and purse straps), $5,300 in cash, and no identification.

Taking advantage of crowds, pickpockets steal hundreds of wallets, purses, and other belongings each year. Women who hang a purse over one shoulder are especially vulnerable if it twists toward her back. Sometimes to create confusion an accomplice will push the emergency stop button, as if by accident, and say, "Oh darn, sorry." Sometimes one pickpocket will engage you in small talk while the other rifles your possessions. And sometimes, working in teams, two or three members will get on the elevator and maneuver you snugly against a team member already present on the elevator.

But no matter what technique the pickpockets utilize on elevators, most thefts can be prevented if you focus on your purse, wallet, etc., and think, Are these secure? Pickpockets are successful because you are not thinking about pickpockets and you are not familiar with their techniques.

People Press

Groups of pickpockets use some version of the "people press." In this technique a group of pickpockets will press against you in a lobby or in the street. Maybe the groups will be asking questions, begging money, singing, or dancing. But the idea is always the same. They are trying to distract and confuse you and push you into a position so they can steal the wallet from your purse or your watch from your wrist. Many times the pickpockets will take advantage of situations in which people are naturally pressed together on elevators, crowded trains, lines for popular movies, and at intersections where crowds are waiting to cross the street.

Baby Bounce

The "baby bounce" is a technique whereby pickpockets use a baby to distract your attention and occupy your arms. Typically a cute young child tugs at the leg of your pants or falls down in front of you. As you lift the child someone may be stealing your possessions. There are many different forms of the baby bounce. A woman in Washington, D.C., told the author she was in a grocery store and noticed a three-year-old girl who was crying and appeared to be separated from her mother. The woman picked up the child and found the mother two aisles away. When the woman returned to her grocery cart she discovered her purse was stolen. It was later discovered that this same child was "lost" in at least seven other stores.

There are, of course, many other versions of the baby bounce technique. Sometimes a man or a woman will ask you to hold their infant while they adjust the baby's stroller, gather packages, or whatever. While you are holding the baby someone picks your pocket or steals the packages you have set down. Even if you feel the person stealing your wallet you cannot just throw the baby down and give chase.

It should also be pointed out that children are often used as stage props. Who would suspect an innocent-looking woman with a beautiful baby to be a pickpocket or shoplifter? Nevertheless, in scores of recorded cases stolen loot has been hidden in a baby's blanket or diaper. If anyone tries to search the mother she begins breast-feeding her baby. Women pushing baby carriages have also been known to surveil neighborhoods for burglars.

Thieves utilize babies and children in many different ways. At Los Angeles International Airport a burly armored car guard was signing for a cash pickup when a two-foot, two-year-old toddler tugged at his trousers and took a money pouch from his hand cart. Attracting little attention, the girl waddled to her father and presented him with $8,500. The single witness to the crime alerted the guard, who quickly caught the father walking away with the cash. But before an arrest could be made, the little girl's mother, acting shocked, handed the cash to the guard and apologized profusely. It all seemed like an innocent and rather funny childish incident until the police decided to surveil the con artist couple. Incredibly, they caught the trio practicing their con with arriving and departing passengers. The child would grab purses from women waiting for flights and even picked up a briefcase from a woman who had placed it on the floor while she signed a rental car agreement.

We certainly are not advising that you avoid cute or lost children. After all, most encounters with children will be perfectly innocent and beautiful. Help the child, appreciate the child, hug the child if you like, but also be street smart and think, "Is this a setup?"

Want to Buy a Ring?

A forty-year-old woman attending a security conference directed by the author explained how she once lost a $15,000 ring that had been in her family for two generations. While shopping in an exclusive area of San Francisco the woman was approached by a man on the sidewalk who offered to sell her a ring. The woman explained that she wasn't interested but the man persisted and displayed a beautiful diamond ring for a very low price. Believing that the ring was probably stolen, the woman again explained that she wasn't interested. But the man still persisted and said, "Just put the ring on your finger and if you still don't want it I'll take it back and leave." Succumbing to the hard sell, the woman agreed and allowed the man to put the ring on her finger. She explained that the ring was beautiful but she still did not want it. Consequently, the man slipped his ring off the woman's finger and departed. A minute later the woman noticed that he had also slipped her $15,000 ring off her finger.

Where Is Your Wallet Located?

If a pickpocket has targeted you he or she may first
want to determine where your wallet is located. Is the
wallet in the outside compartment of your purse? Is
the wallet in your briefcase? Most frequently the pickpocket determines the location of your wallet by ob-
serving where you place it after making a purchase.
Sometimes the bulge in your pocket signals the wallet's location. But frequently a pickpocket will use a
trick or a ruse to determine the location of your wallet.
Perhaps a friendly person will approach you with a
ten-dollar bill and ask if you have change. You pull
your wallet from your left coat pocket to give the
person change and that person now knows the wallet's
location. Frequently a pickpocket will approach you
with a wallet partially concealed in his hand and say,
"Excuse me, miss, did you lose your wallet?" Instinc-
tively you pat your pocket or check your purse to
make sure you still have your wallet—and the pickpocket now knows its location. One trick for locating
your wallet is over 100 years old. At strategic locations
thieves would post large signs that stated, Beware of
Pickpockets. People would see these signs and immediately pat their pockets to make sure their wallets
were still there. The pickpockets would watch the people pat their pockets and know where the wallet was
located.

Once the pickpocketing team determines where
your wallet is located they may "accidentally" bump
into you two blocks down the street, "dance" with
you on an escalator, or squirt ketchup on your blouse.

Thefts From Rest Rooms

Thieves notoriously target rest rooms. One favored tactic is to reach over the bathroom stall and steal the purse or coat (which often has a wallet in the pocket) from the inside hook. Naturally, any items left outside the booth when you are using the toilet are easy pickings for a thief. A lot of purses and shoulder bags turn up missing when women are using mirrors in crowded bathrooms, especially in airports. Also, a purse left on the floor inside a stall can be easily grabbed from the front or from a stall next to you.

Increasingly, female pickpockets are posing as bathroom attendants. With an easily obtained uniform the fake attendant waits in the bathroom with a towel over one arm as a prop, and a plate of coins (tips) to her side. You walk in, hand your belongings to the attendant to hold, and she walks out with your possessions. This tactic has most frequently been reported in fancy hotels.

Taxis

Always watch a taxi driver load all your luggage into the trunk of the car and wait until he closes the trunk before entering the backseat. Some dishonest taxi drivers will purposely leave one bag outside the trunk, which is picked up by a criminal accomplice. If there is more than one passenger, make sure that she or he doesn't accidentally or purposely take any of your bags if she/he gets out first. In one case known to the author the taxi driver and the other "passenger" were in cahoots and stole dozens of bags using this technique.

Be polite but do not offer the taxi driver too much

information about yourself. Hundreds of crimes of all types have been traced back to information supplied to a taxi driver. Remember, if he is taking you to a hotel or to your home or office he already knows where you are staying. Some women, uncomfortable with questions asked by taxi drivers, have been dropped off a block from their residence so the driver wouldn't know where they live.

Never accept food, candy, or drink from a taxi driver; it might be spiked with a drug that puts you to sleep. Refuse even if he offers you a cookie and states, innocently, "My wife baked these for my birthday, please help me celebrate." Women drugged by taxi drivers have been robbed and raped.

Guard Your Valuables

The wife and three-year-old daughter of a Japanese businessman landed at an international airport in the United States after visiting relatives in Tokyo. As might be expected after such a long trip, the woman was hot and tired and the child was restless. Carrying the child in one arm, the woman piled her luggage on a cart, endured a long line at customs, and finally exited the airport. The woman was relieved to see that a female friend of the family was parked and waiting for her curbside. After waving exuberantly to the driver, the woman deposited her luggage on the side-walk, walked about ten feet to the car, and handed her child to her friend. The woman returned to the side-walk for her luggage and was immediately overcome with a sick feeling of desperation. Someone had stolen her purse and shoulder bag! The woman had turned her back for one minute and someone ran off with her expensive Gucci purse and shoulder bag containing passports, personal papers, house keys, glasses, telephone directory, jewelry, and $4,800 in cash.

Wearing Expensive Watches and Jewelry

A woman who wears expensive watches and jewelry dramatically increases the chances she will be targeted, followed, and mugged. In today's world of violence and crime, if a woman wears a Rolex or Piaget watch she might as well be walking down the street with thousands of dollars in cash strapped conspicuously to her wrist.

The typical scenario is reenacted over and over again. The criminal spots a woman with expensive jewelry and decides to follow her to her home, hotel, or office, waiting for an opportune time to attack. Now he or she knows where the woman lives or works and can choose to attack now or later.

In one case reported to the author a woman was followed home from an exclusive shopping district by a man who noticed her fine diamond necklace and earrings. When the woman got out of her car in her driveway the gunman stole her earrings, necklace, watch, and purse. Grabbing her keys, he ordered her into her house, where she was beaten, raped, and tied while the man burglarized the home. The man then loaded valuable household items into the woman's car and drove away. So this woman was originally targeted for her jewelry but ended up being beaten, raped, and robbed of her jewelry, purse, car, and other items.

A woman who told the author she was not worried about her jewelry "because it is insured" failed to comprehend the domino effect of crime. Women targeted for their jewelry have been wounded and murdered in every state and every country.

An Oklahoma killer who has since been executed entered a home looking for expensive jewelry known to belong to one of the female residents and ended up murdering two women and a man. A niece of Senator Abraham Ribicoff, a twenty-three-year-old graduate of Yale, was murdered in the streets of Venice, California, for her gold chain necklace. A New Jersey woman was attacked by a man who struck her in the head with a brick, knocking her to the ground. When she tried to fight the man off, he slashed her with a knife and removed her gold necklace.

Incredibly, tens of thousands of women have similar stories to tell. Sophia Loren, Zsa Zsa Gabor, and Georgette Mosbacher, cosmetics executive and wife of the former secretary of commerce, were all robbed of jewelry at gunpoint. An heiress was robbed four times over a nine-year period, losing approximately $13 million worth of jewelry! In one incident she was abducted from New York's La Guardia Airport and lost $1 million worth of jewelry.

After being robbed at knife point in her own home, she was quoted as saying, "I'm switching to costume jewelry and I think everyone else should, too." The problem, of course, is that most street thugs are not sophisticated enough to determine if it's costume or real jewelry.

Statistically, most women will wear jewelry their entire lives and never have a problem. Nevertheless, the same criminal statistics clearly indicate that several thousand women will be victimized every year simply because they are wearing gold, silver, and diamonds. There is no question that if a woman wears an expensive watch and jewelry she increases the overall security risk.

Purse Snatchers

In Los Angeles, an older woman was murdered by a would-be purse snatcher in a busy supermarket parking lot. After leaving the supermarket at nine A.M., she was confronted by a man who tried to tear her purse from her grip. When she resisted, the purse snatcher produced a handgun and severely beat her on the head. The man fled to a waiting car without the purse. The victim was pronounced dead one hour later.

Drugged and desperate criminals in the United States and throughout the world are increasingly walking, running, biking, or driving up to women and stealing their purses.

Commonly referred to as "purse snatching," this criminal occupation relies little on finesse and greatly on opportunity, speed, and violence.

Unlike pickpockets, who rarely hurt their targets, purse snatchers frequently leave their targets badly injured or, in dozens of cases, dead.

Many victims, especially older women, have received broken bones and severe head injuries when purse snatchers have shoved them to the sidewalk or street. Many muggers cut purse straps with a sharp knife, often slicing skin as well. A few women have been dragged beneath vehicles and killed when criminals in passing cars have grabbed their purses. In these cases the women had apparently wrapped the purse strap around their wrists to prevent it from being pulled away.

A woman was dragged by a train in New York and killed while chasing a man who had snatched her purse. Shortly after the train pulled from the station a man grabbed her purse and ran. Although she had only one dollar in her purse, she chased the mugger until she slipped between the car and the platform, breaking many major bones and nearly severing her left leg. She bled to death chasing a purse snatcher.

Scores of men have been wounded or killed while rushing to the rescue of their wives and girlfriends. A doctor was shot to death in Brooklyn when he tried to prevent a mugger from stealing his wife's purse. The doctor and his wife were returning from a dinner party at eleven P.M., and had just parked their car when a man approached them from the front and without saying a word grabbed the wife's purse. She held on to her purse and her husband grabbed it as well. The mugger pulled a handgun and shot the doctor in the chest.

In purse snatchings, as with most crimes, innocent bystanders are frequently killed. In Philadelphia, two men spotted two women as they left a restaurant and slowly followed them in their car. One of the men, now out of the car, walked up to one of the women and snatched her purse as she was sorting through one of its compartments. The purse snatcher then ran back to his car and the two men sped away. In their haste to escape, the two men ran a stop sign, hit another car, and ran up on a sidewalk, killing a young innocent bystander.

With serial murderers on the loose and headlines filled with gruesome crimes against women, purse snatchers are often relegated to mere nuisance status. But thousands of women in the United States know better. Purse snatchings are frequently very violent.

A review of hundreds of incidents suggests that women are most vulnerable when they are carrying their purse in a lazy, haphazard manner, when they appear inattentive or preoccupied, and when their body language communicates a disregard for personal security and personal space. If someone thinks, It can't happen to me, it shows!

Women who wrap their purse strap around their

wrist to prevent theft have frequently been pulled down and dragged by purse snatchers. When one nervous purse snatcher finally pulled a gun and screamed at a woman to "let go!" she couldn't, because the strap was tied to her wrist. Some of the most serious injuries have occurred when women put the strap over their neck; the strap works as a garrotte when yanked by the purse snatcher. Also, seeing that the strap will get hung up on the woman's neck, many muggers will cut the strap and often the skin beneath as well.

Although some women have struggled with purse snatchers and hung on long enough to discourage their efforts, the highest percentage of beatings, knifings, and shootings occurred when the woman (or husband/boyfriend) either fought back or gave chase.

Being aware of the purse-snatching threat, women are cradling their purses close to their bodies, guarding their personal space and increasingly communicating an alert, street-smart attitude.

Distractions and Diversions

In a very high percentage of all pickpocketings and bag thefts the criminals utilize some form of distraction or diversion. Sometimes the distraction is devised or staged by the criminal ("Do you have change for twenty dollars?") and sometimes the criminals rely on "natural" distractions. A woman carrying groceries and trying to put her children in the car is a good example of someone who is naturally distracted. The criminal knows that when we are distracted we are more vulnerable. Consequently, it is important to know what these "staged" and "natural" distractions are and to think security when we are in those situations.

In a study of almost 10,000 cases in which people

lost wallets, purses, briefcases, etc., to pickpockets
and sneak thieves, the author identified the most commonly used distractions and diversions, staged and
natural. It should be pointed out that some of these
distractions—someone asking directions or someone
asking for the time—have been utilized tens of thousands of times, not only by pickpockets, but by rapists, kidnappers, muggers, etc. In other words, a tactic
used by pickpockets may also be used by rapists and
murderers. Knowledge of these distractions is part of
being street smart and can give you that split-second
advantage that may save your purse—or your life.

STAGED DISTRACTIONS

The most common *staged* distractions are as follows:

1. "Can you tell me how to get to . . . ?" Criminals
    on foot or in a car frequently *ask for directions* as
    a way to distract you or bring you within reach.
    This has been used *thousands* of times by pick-
    pockets, child molesters, rapists, serial murder-
    ers, and others. On the one hand we need to be
    cautious, but on the other hand we need to help
    our fellow citizens and visitors. (Most people
    who ask directions are genuinely lost!) Conse-
    quently, when someone asks for directions keep
    a distance, politely and quickly respond if you
    choose, but at the same time be aware of what is
    around you and think, Is this a setup? Consider
    the following cases: (a) A woman walking in
    Silver Spring, Maryland, was approached by a
    man asking directions. When the woman turned
    to point the way, the man knocked her down and
    stole her purse. (b) In Huntington Beach, Cali-
    fornia, a woman was walking to her car parked
    near her apartment, when two men asked for

directions. The woman was kidnapped and raped. (c) In Orange County, Florida, a fifteen-year-old girl was abducted by a man who asked for directions and pulled her into his van.

2. "Can you tell me the time?" This too is a question that is normally innocent but should set off warning signals; thousands of pickpockets, rapists, robbers, etc., have used it as a tactic. Often criminals just want to get you to look at your watch for a couple of seconds while they make their move. Keep your distance, be aware of what's behind you, respond on the move. Consider the following cases: (a) Runner Shelley Reecher (mentioned in "Attacks on Joggers") was dragged into a car and raped by four men, who had asked for the time. (b) A fourteen-year-old girl in Fairfax, Virginia, was pulled into the woods near her school and raped by a man who had called her over and asked for the time. (c) A man tried to abduct a forty-four-year-old Springfield, Virginia, woman from a library parking lot after asking her for the time. Remember, many thieves will ask for the time just to see if you are wearing an expensive watch.

3. Pickpockets will frequently "accidentally" bump into you as a distraction.

4. Pickpockets, sneak thieves, and others will often stage a loud argument or fake a fight as a distraction.

5. A thief holding a notebook may ask you for a pen. A thief holding a cigarette may ask you for a light.

6. A person or group of people may drop a cup of coins on the floor as a distraction.

7. As a diversion someone may suddenly approach you with a lot of questions. (They will usually try to get right up to your face.)

8. "Could you hold my baby, please?"

9. Be suspicious of someone overly eager to be helpful.

10. Be suspicious of someone who persistently steps in front of you and tries to sell you something. Is he trying to block your view from something? Is his accomplice behind you?

11. Be extremely leery of street-corner opinion and educational surveys, especially sexual question-naires. "Hi, I'm a psychology student conduct-ing a study on . . ." Don't be naive! Some so-called studies have been conducted by sex of-fenders trying to obtain personal information on future targets. Some women have unwittingly volunteered information that has hurt them-selves and others.

12. Don't overreact but be cautious if someone spills a drink on you or mentions that you have ketchup on your clothes.

NATURAL DISTRACTIONS

Pickpockets, sneak thieves, and purse snatchers also rely on so-called natural distractions. In fact, these criminals will frequently stake out areas where people will be naturally distracted in airports, shopping malls, hotels, and so forth. Ten of the most common natural distractions are as follows:

1. A hurried businesswoman holding several pieces of luggage and trying to decipher the arrival/departure screen at a busy airport is naturally distracted.

2. A woman carrying groceries and trying to mind children at the same time is naturally distracted and often has her purse stolen by a pickpocket or purse snatcher when she lifts a small child into the backseat.

3. A woman hailing a taxi or paying a taxi is naturally distracted. She often puts her briefcase on the sidewalk, fumbles through her purse for money, and leans back inside the taxi to pay the driver. At that point her briefcase on the sidewalk is unguarded. Pay the driver before you get out of the taxi.

4. A person watching the luggage conveyor belt at an airport and wrestling with the ubiquitous crowd is naturally distracted. Frequently we will set our carry-on luggage down (unattended) and then push through the crowd to get our checked luggage.

5. When you are using a pay phone you are naturally distracted in many ways. (See "Security at Pay Telephones.") Women are extremely vulnerable to many different types of crimes at pay phones.

6. A woman pushing a grocery cart and preoccupied with reaching food on a top shelf is naturally distracted. Hundreds of purses are stolen from grocery stores each year.

7. When you are signing a rental-car agreement at an airport, your briefcase and luggage are an easy target. You are tired, facing away from your bags, and concentrating on the contract.

8. Many women have reported bags stolen when they were checking in or checking out at the front desk of a hotel.

9. Anytime you are fiddling for your keys, carrying bundles, and searching for your car in a crowded parking lot you are vulnerable. Have your keys ready, remember exactly where you are parked, and concentrate on what and who is around you.

10. Women are often targeted by purse snatchers and pickpockets while walking and fumbling with an umbrella and holding their skirts down on wet and windy days.

REDUCING THE RISK

1. The most effective weapon we have against pickpockets and bag snatchers is *knowledge of their tactics*. A street-smart woman aware of the ketchup squirt, the crumpled money trick, the escalator dance, and so on is less likely to be a victim of those tactics. If you are familiar with *staged* and *natural* distractions you are less likely to be caught off guard and more likely to make wise security decisions.

2. A number of security companies produce small, portable alarms that emit ear-piercing sounds if you are personally attacked or if your possessions are moved or pulled from you. The personal attack alarms, about the size of a standard beeper,

can be easily and quickly activated by you in case of attack. Personal property-protection alarms attach to your purse, briefcase, etc. If someone pulls your purse away from you the alarm sounds automatically; the thief will be running with a loud alarm coming out of your purse. Property-protection motion-detector alarms can also be attached to *unattended* briefcases, ski boots, bicycles, etc. If your property is moved, the ear-piercing alarm sounds. A loud noise is an excellent deterrent to crime.

3. If you fall asleep on a train or bus, or while waiting for a flight, thieves will consider you an easy target. Try to maintain contact with your possessions. Increasingly, people are even tying briefcases and purses to the seat or their person when they feel sleepy.

4. A woman who wears expensive jewelry and watches dramatically increases the chances she will be targeted by muggers and thieves. Remember, one crime often leads to many other crimes. In hundreds of recorded cases women targeted for their jewelry were also abducted, raped, wounded, or killed.

5. A handbag dangling loosely from a woman's shoulder or elbow is a tempting target for a pickpocket or purse snatcher. Be sure your handbag can be securely closed. Keep the wallet deep inside the bag, preferably in a zippered compartment. If possible, put your purse strap under your coat. Women who put the purse across their neck risk being choked. Women who wrap the purse strap several times around their wrists risk being dragged. Never just hang a purse over a chair; it's

too easy to grab. Remember, hundreds of purses and coats have been grabbed from the inside hook in a toilet stall. Divide your valuables between pockets, wallet, handbag, etc. In other words, don't put all your valuables in one place. Consider using a "fanny pack" or a money belt. If you are wearing slacks and socks, an ankle wallet (secured to your ankle with Velcro and worn under a sock) is considered very safe from pickpockets and muggers. Do not lay your purse down while shopping. Many women carry an empty purse as a decoy and carry money, credit cards, and identification hidden on their person.

6. Step one in a criminal setup may be a simple question like, "Do you have the time?" "Do you have change?" "How do I get to . . . ?" A wide variety of pickpockets, purse snatchers, rapists, and serial murderers have used these setups to distract your attention, draw you near, and catch you off guard. If approached with these questions, answer on the move (move back or away, not forward), be aware of who is behind you, and, if you choose to respond, answer politely and quickly. Ask yourself, "Could this be a setup?" and do not be afraid to be impolite.

7. Thousands of purse snatchings and mugging incidents that turned violent suggest that you will reduce the risk if you do not fight, grab, or resist. Remember, many muggers do not display a weapon until they meet with resistance and a mugger that appears to be alone may be working with an armed backup or lookout. Too many fighters overlook the lookout. Yes, there is a time to fight. And when you fight you "go animal"; no squeamishness, no mercy allowed. You bite and

rip a nose; you viciously claw an eye; you kick, knee, and grab a groin. You fight to win. But in this case you are losing a purse, not a child. The decision to fight is always up to the individual (the experts are home watching television), but that decision to fight should be based on survival, not anger or ego; on reason, not panic. You do not risk it all for a purse or briefcase. And you have to make a decision whether you want your mate to risk it all. Chivalry is not dead and many men, if threatened, will fight on impulse, partly out of instinct and partly because they feel that you (the woman) expect it! Therefore, it is important to discuss with your husband/boyfriend your fight/flight philosophy. If you don't want him to risk it all for a purse, tell him so!

Be willing to give up a small battle to win the war. And remember, if it comes down to survival, if your instincts say you must "go for it," understand you are ten times stronger and more vicious than you ever imagined.

8. Knockout drugs, or "Mickey Finns," designed to put you to sleep or render you helpless, are used at least 900 times per month in the United States. Ten years ago these drugs were used primarily by prostitutes who would put their male clients to sleep and steal their Rolex watches. Today, two things are different: (a) Knockout drugs are being used by a wide variety of criminals, including serial murderers, rapists, child molesters, etc. (b) Increasingly, knockout drugs are being used on women. This trend is going to increase. Do not accept food, drink, or candy from strangers—the same advice we have given our children for years. If you are in an uncomfortable or suspicious situation with a male or female you don't know or

trust, don't give that person the opportunity to use this tactic. Just as knockout drugs have been used to steal jewelry and wallets from men, the same tactic will increasingly be used on women. Do not leave your drink unattended when you go to the rest room. Be very careful when a stranger (man or woman) introduces himself and hands you a drink. Remember, you are most vulnerable when you are alone and/or drinking.

12

Crime in the Home Environment

Several million murders, assaults, rapes, arsons, burglaries, and other crimes occur at private homes and apartments each year in the United States.

In 1991 there were 3.2 million *reported* burglaries in the United States—and burglary is only one of several types of crime that occur in the home environment. Approximately 70 percent of these burglaries involved forced entry (breaking a window, knocking a lock off a door, etc.) and about 60 percent of the total burglaries occurred during the daylight hours.

Increasingly, a wide variety of brazen, drugged, and desperate criminals are more willing to enter homes and offices while people are present. In fact, during 1991, approximately 480,000 homes were entered by criminals while at least one member of the family was actually in the house. In 1991 at least 144,000 burglaries resulted in at least one family member being murdered, wounded, raped, or violently attacked.

Approximately 800,000 burglaries would have been

prevented in 1991 if the victims had simply locked their doors and windows.

Tens of thousands of other crimes in the home environment would have been prevented if the victims had practiced better security and had a better awareness of criminal tactics, ruses, and disguises.

The following sections are designed to increase your security awareness and to help save lives, property, and money.

Make Your Home Look Occupied

One of the most effective deterrents to crime is to make your home appear to be occupied. Leaving some lights on—and perhaps a radio or television—will persuade many criminal opportunists to move on. If you are going to be away for a while, stop your mail and newspaper deliveries or have a trusted friend pick these up. When mail or newspapers accumulate, it signals to criminals that you and your family are away. Consider replacing your outside mailbox with an in-door mail slot. There are two reasons for this: (a) visible mail signals vacancy; (b) mail in a mailbox is easily stolen and can be utilized by a variety of criminals. If you go on vacation it is also important to have someone mow your lawn and shovel your snow. Long grass and unshoveled snow signals vacancy to a criminal.

Consider purchasing light timers that will automatically turn various lights in your home on and off at different times. Light timers have certainly fooled many potential burglars and can be purchased for a reasonable price. It should be remembered, however, that most break-ins occur during the day, when most lights are off. Furthermore, many criminals will simply knock at your door to determine if someone is home.

Lock Your Doors and Windows

The statistics clearly show that it is very important to lock your doors and windows when you are home and when you are away from home. More than 800,000 homes and offices were burglarized in the United States during 1991 simply because someone left a door or window unlocked. In other words, in 800,000 burglaries, the criminal did not smash a window or place a gun to the owner's head; he or she simply walked in through an unlocked window or door, stole valuables, and walked out. But there are much more important reasons for locking your doors and windows. In 1991 nearly 35,000 people were murdered, raped, or injured by criminals who gained access through an unlocked door or window.

It takes very little time and effort to lock up. Today tens of thousands of victims are saying to themselves, "I wish I had locked that door."

When securing your home, priority number one is to obtain proper door and window locks. Many new homes are supplied with the cheapest locks the builder could find, so it behooves you to upgrade your security hardware. The installation of strong door and window locks is one of the least expensive but most important security precautions you can implement.

Basically, there are three components to a secure door: the door itself, the locks, and the jamb, which is the side post of the doorway. If any of these three components is weak, it won't matter that the other two components are strong. Security, like a chain, is only as strong as its weakest link.

DOORS

1. The DOOR—An entry door should be solid-core (not hollow) and contain as little glass as possible. If you must have a decorative window it should have metal grilles or be upgraded to a polycarbon or other difficult-to-break glass. Hinge pins should be on the inside so the burglar cannot remove them. Studies have shown that burglars most frequently enter through a back door that is usually hidden from the street and out of neighbors' view.

2. THE LOCKS—Most experts recommend a strong, good-quality deadbolt for important entry doors. Key-in-knob-type locks (locks that are on the doorknob) are weak and easy to defeat. A deadbolt works by sending a bolt from the lock on the door to the jamb. The deadbolt should have a throw (the extension of the bolt past the door) of at least one inch. Rather than replacing your original lock, it is usually easier and more effective to simply add an auxiliary deadbolt.

3. THE DOORJAMB—Criminals know that the jamb is often the weakest link and the most frequently overlooked. It doesn't matter that the door and locks are strong if the whole apparatus is attached to something weak. It is important to reinforce the strike plate, the plate through which the bolt passes in the jamb. The strike plate should be secured in solid wood with four-inch screws.

Most experts do not have much confidence in door chain locks, which allow you to open a door a few inches to see who is on the other side. The reason they don't have confidence is because in many cases attackers have simply shoved their shoulder against the door and yanked the chain and its screws from the jamb. However, when high-quality chain locks are properly reinforced by a professional, such devices certainly add another dimension to your security.

Rather than a chain lock, however, it is better to install a wide-angle viewer (a peephole) in the door. This way you simply look through the peephole and don't have to open the door at all.

WINDOWS

Following the back door, burglars and other criminals most frequently enter through first-floor and basement windows. Since windows are primarily made of glass, they are easy to break and enter. Breaking the glass, however, usually makes noise, so most burglars prefer to jimmy the window locks.

Double-hung windows come with a variety of locks but most are undependable and easy to defeat. To counter this weakness we suggest the following procedure: (a) Drill a small hole where the windows overlap when closed. (b) Insert a nail or screw in the hole. This will make it very difficult for a burglar to pull the window open. Do not drill the hole all the way through both windows (if you do, the burglar can simply push the screw or nail out). Drill the hole at a slight downward angle so the nail/screw can't be tapped out. When you want to open the window yourself, just remove the nail or screw.

Burglary statistics clearly illustrate that basement windows are extremely vulnerable. (Tens of thousands of burglars have entered residences through the basement window.) Here we have a number of options: (a) Put a strong metal grate or grille over the window. (b) Put a deadbolt lock on the door that leads from the basement to the first floor. If there is no grille on the window but a deadbolt lock on the door, the criminal can enter the basement but cannot gain access to living quarters of the house. (c) Install metal grilles on the basement windows *and* install a deadbolt lock on the basement door. Obviously, the deadbolt should not be installed on the basement side of the door where the burglar would have access to the mechanism.

Statistically, sliding patio doors are also extremely vulnerable. They have notoriously weak locks and are easy to derail. Sliding glass patio doors are normally divided into two halves. One half is stationary and the other half slides back and forth. For about ten dollars you can purchase a special metal bar that will immobilize the sliding section of the door, even if the door is unlocked.

Unfortunately, many desperate criminals are quite willing to make noise and break glass in order to gain entry. Consequently, if you desire extra security you will have to install metal grates or bars over your windows and glass patio doors or replace the glass with break-resistant polycarbon plastic panes. Remember, bars on windows certainly keep burglars out but they can also be dangerous to you. In case of fire, bars on windows may prevent you from exiting through a window or may prevent a fireman from entering through a window. Consequently, if you install bars on windows, install them on the inside of the window and choose the type that can be removed or swung open in case of fire. With this type of removable bar you need to be sure the key is readily available on a hook next to the window. You don't want to be searching for a key when there's a fire.

Also remember, if you forget to lock your doors and windows, all the locks, alarms, and metal grilles in the world will not help you!

REDUCING THE RISK

1. Don't give a burglar a place to hide. Bushes and shrubbery near the house should be trimmed so a burglar can't hide while he works on your window.

2. Outdoor lights are very effective in discouraging a burglar. Criminals do not want to be spotlighted while they work.

3. Don't leave garden tools or ladders in the yard. Many burglars, rapists, and even child kidnappers have utilized ladders to gain access to second-floor rooms. Garden tools can be used to pry open doors and windows. Since criminals don't want to be caught with burglary tools, many will use only tools they find in the yard.

4. Don't hide your key under your doormat or in your mailbox; the criminal will look in those places. If you hide a house key it should be well hidden several steps from the front door.

5. If someone knocks at your door and claims to be selling something or claims to have the wrong address, be suspicious. He or she might be trying to determine if anyone is home. Observe where the person goes next and try to get a license plate number if he or she has a car.

6. Remember, burglars and other criminals come in all ages, including the very young and the very old. In addition, they have pretended to be priests and nuns, police officers, flower-delivery personnel, telephone repairmen, etc.

7. Don't forget to lock your garage. Once inside the garage the burglar can work unnoticed on the door leading to your family. In addition, various criminals will hide in the garage and ambush the homeowner.

8. If you enjoy pets consider getting a dog. Dogs have been guarding humans since time began. University researchers who have interviewed hundreds of incarcerated criminals have concluded that criminals tend to avoid homes with dogs. If you don't want a dog consider putting a Beware of Dog sign in your yard and a huge dog dinner bowl on your front porch. For added drama put a creative name on the bowl. Some people have named their fictitious dogs "Killer," "Fang," "Dobby the Doberman," and "Dinosaur." Some alarm companies even sell tapes of angry dogs barking. If you are away from the house the tape will "bark" every few minutes.

9. If you cannot afford an alarm system an alarm decal will be effective in discouraging many criminals. Many burglars say they can usually tell if a decal genuinely represents an alarm system, but they figure, Why take the chance?

10. Consider putting valuable computers, stereos, etc., away from windows. This way if a burglar looks in he'll think you are not worth the effort.

11. Secure valuables in place. Televisions, stereos and other valuables that are rarely moved can be secured with small screws. You are not trying to bolt them down permanently but only trying to reduce their "grabability." The idea is to make it more difficult for the burglar to operate quickly.

12. Think of creative places to hide jewelry and other valuables. Burglars are in a hurry and are frequently intoxicated or drugged. They don't have much patience with hide-and-seek. Warning: Don't forget where the items are hidden and tell a family member in case you die unexpectedly. Don't be too creative! The author's friend hid diamonds in frozen ice-cube trays. This trick certainly fooled a burglar who broke into the house on Christmas Eve, but on New Year's Day her father sipped on a cocktail and swallowed a diamond ring. Fortunately, the ring was returned twenty-four hours later, but her father didn't enjoy the search!

13. If you have reason to believe that an intruder is in your home when you return, *do not enter*. If a vehicle is parked on or near your property, get a description and a license plate number and call the police or have a neighbor do so. Dial 911 and report "burglary in progress" at your address. Don't try to be a hero. Cornered burglars are dangerous animals who frequently shoot in panic.

⬡ 13

The Postal Ploy

In the exciting movie *Three Days of the Condor**
starring Robert Redford, an assassin dons a mailman's uniform, rings the doorbell of his intended victim, and claims to have a special-delivery package.
Offering to sign for the package, Malcolm, the target,
asks the mailman if he has a pen. "The mailman
slapped his pockets unsuccessfully." "Come on in,"
Malcolm said. "I'll get one." When Malcolm went
into the kitchen to find a pen the mailman pulled a
silenced submachine gun out of his pouch. . . .

Since that movie came out, fiction has become fact
on scores of occasions. Criminals and terrorists in the
United States have posed as postmen and committed
a long series of murders, home invasions, rapes, robberies, and kidnappings. And each victim, taken by
surprise, was wide-eyed with shock when the mailman
turned out to be a criminal.

Malcolm, the hero in *Three Days of the Condor,*

---

*Based on the book *Six Days of the Condor* by James Grady.

panicked when he heard the doorbell ring. But then, "He sighed with relief when he saw through the one-way glass peephole that it was only a bored-looking mailman, his bag slung over one shoulder, a package in one hand."

Hundreds of real-life victims have also made the mistake of concluding, "He's just a mailman." Consider the following real-life cases in which women were targeted:

A man wearing an official postal uniform rang the doorbell at a home in Maryland. A woman who was baby-sitting for a small child answered the door. "Special-delivery package," said the postman. The baby-sitter opened the door a few inches but the chain and lock were still attached. "You'll have to open the door, ma'am, and sign for the package," said the postman, who held out a pen and clipboard. The woman complied with the request and was handed the clipboard and pen. As she signed for the package the phony postman and another man who had been hiding pushed their way into the house and pulled out handguns. The robbers tied the woman with rope and locked her in a bathroom. They then carried the little boy from the upstairs bedroom to the basement bathroom and ransacked the home, looking for valuables.

The men stole a handgun, cash, and other valuables and fled the scene. About one hour later the woman was able to work her hands loose and freed herself from the bathroom. The child was traumatized but not injured.

In Miami, Florida, a woman was shot to death when a man posing as a United Parcel Service deliveryman and a female partner burst into her home. It was the second time in a week someone committed a home invasion dressed in a UPS uniform.

A cleaning woman in the victim's home heard a knock at the door, looked out the window, and saw a man in a UPS uniform. A savvy former crime victim, the cleaning woman, quoted in the local paper, stated, "I didn't see the UPS truck. That's what made me so nervous and upset."

Her employer, who apparently didn't heed the cleaning woman's warnings, unlocked the door. The door was open about six inches when the fake UPS man, followed by a female accomplice, pushed their way inside.

Apparently intending robbery, the man and woman initially encountered the woman's young male relative, who responded to the commotion. The man was shot in the head and was seriously wounded. Showing no mercy, the disguised duo then turned their guns on the woman, ending her life.

Criminals have obtained postal uniforms in many different ways. In some cases the uniforms were stolen from homes, cars, and dry cleaners or simply purchased from private uniform stores or pawnshops. In other cases the uniforms were obtained from former postal employees. The bottom line is that postal uniforms are not difficult to obtain.

REDUCING THE RISK

1. Since real postmen show up every day you obviously need to assess the circumstances before raising eyebrows in suspicion. How frequently does the real postman knock at your door? What time does the real postman usually arrive? One woman failed to be suspicious when the "postman" arrived at night; another failed to be suspicious when the "postman" arrived on Sunday. Do you recognize this guy or is he new? If you have suspicions don't open the door.

2. Postal officials say to look for a badge or an identification card. True, any identification can be stolen or forged but most impostors of record relied on the uniform alone.

3. Are you expecting a "special delivery"? Ask questions. Who is it from? It's very suspicious when the package doesn't have a return address. Is there any postage on the package? It's very suspicious when there is too much postage, too little postage, or no postage at all. Does the form you are signing look official?

4. Is there a postal Jeep or truck parked outside? In many cases the impostors had no visible means of transportation; in one case the "postman" reportedly showed up in a Corvette! Remember, in some cases impostors have stolen official postal Jeeps.

5. Take a look at the uniform. Sometimes the impostors only steal the top portion of the uniform; do the slacks match? Statistically, if one part of the impostor's uniform (whether it be postmen, policemen, or whatever) is inappropriate, it's usually the shoes. Impostors will usually steal uniforms but they stick with their own shoes. Learn to be observant. It's odd when someone is wearing a working man's uniform with coat and tie shoes.

6. Be very cautious if a postman you don't recognize asks for a glass of water or asks to use the bathroom or telephone.

7. An age-old trick of phony deliverymen and phony postmen, etc., is to claim their pen is out of ink. "Do you have a pen?" The strategy here is that you will turn your back, leave the door

open, and leave to get a pen. When you return the impostor is in the house.

8. If you're alone in the house there's nothing wrong with a little theatrics. Before opening the door yell, loud enough for the caller to hear, "I'll get it, honey." Heck, go ahead and have some fun! Yell, "George, hold the dogs, someone is at the front door." (But there's such a thing as overacting: "George, can't you stop cleaning that shotgun long enough to get the door!")

9. Learn to look for weapons. If that person has a weapon, where could it be concealed? Keep an eye on the hands. Keep in mind that in fiction and real life weapons have been concealed in mailbags.

10. Learn to be observant and attentive to detail. It's not only great for security, it makes life more fun!

14

"May I Use Your Telephone?"

One summer afternoon, a man rang a doorbell at a fashionable home in Pennsylvania. When an eleven-year-old girl who lives in the house responded to the doorbell, the man politely asked, "May I use your telephone please?" The little girl did not know the man but felt it would be impolite to say no. "OK, come on in," she said, "the telephone is in the bedroom." After using the telephone, the man engaged in casual conversation with the little girl, and then suddenly grabbed her from behind and carried her outside. Screaming and kicking, the girl struggled free as the would-be kidnapper tried to stuff her inside his car. When the girl ran back to her house the man quickly drove away.

As a tactic to gain entry to homes, apartments, and offices a wide range of criminals, including serial murderers and rapists, have won the confidence of their victims and defeated security simply by asking, "May I use your telephone?" In fact, the startling reality is that, over the years, *thousands* of women of all ages have been raped, robbed, kidnapped, or murdered by criminals who relied on this one very simple tactic. The tragedy of this finding is obvious; thousands of heinous crimes would have been prevented if the victims had (a) been informed about the "May I use your telephone" ruse and (b) practiced a few simple security precautions.

The author has been informed of over ninety cases in which the "May I use your telephone" tactic has been utilized to commit rapes. In Boston, a man walked into a medical clinic, asked to use the telephone, and brutally raped a lab technician; in Baltimore, a man politely asked to use the telephone and raped a sixty-one-year-old homeowner in her kitchen; in Los Angeles, a man complained of car trouble, asked to use the phone, and raped a twenty-year-old woman in her apartment.

Sadly, many of these ninety-plus rape victims have been children. In Oregon, a ten-year-old girl and her eight-year-old sister were left alone in their home for an hour while their mother went to a health club to work out. The mother was gone only five minutes when a man knocked at the door stating, "My car is broken down, may I use your telephone?" Before departing the man pulled a gun, ordered the young girls into a bathroom, and forced them to take their clothes off. Both girls were sexually assaulted. When their mother arrived home fifty-five minutes later she was naturally horrified to find the front door wide open, the telephone lines severed, and her two weeping daughters huddled in the bathroom.

Although this tactic has been used thousands of times, victims continue to sob, "Nobody ever told me . . . if I had only known." A young girl or a woman aware of a tactic is less likely to become a victim of that tactic.

In Virginia, three teenaged boys knocked at an

apartment door and asked to use the telephone. A teenage girl, who was alone in the apartment, noticed that the boys were about her age and let them in. When one of the boys opened a bedroom door the girl asked him to "please close the door." Instead, the three boys grabbed the girl and forced her onto the bed. While two boys held her down, the third ripped her clothes off and attempted to rape her. Fortunately, in the midst of the attack, the girl's uncle arrived at the apartment, and the assailants fled.

Incredibly, *scores* of women have been either severely wounded or murdered after falling for some version of the "May I use your telephone" tactic. In a high percentage of these cases the criminals claimed one of three reasons for needing the phone: (a) "My car is broken down and I need to call a tow truck." (b) "There's been an accident, I need to call an ambulance." (c) "My phone is out of order, may I use yours?"

Many of the criminals using this tactic have proven to be convincing actors and masters of deception. One such criminal went to a home in Charlotte, North Carolina, woke the two female residents at three A.M. and screamed that his wife had been badly hurt. "Please, please, I need to call a doctor!" he said in a panicky voice. Once inside, the man, who was high on cocaine, grabbed a butcher knife and attacked the two women. One woman received multiple stab wounds and died. Her roommate was stabbed repeatedly but survived. The attacker was executed.

In Florida, a woman was working in her yard when she was approached by a man. "May I use your telephone, please," he said. This was a tactic that had worked well for him in the past. "Of course," the victim is believed to have responded, "I'll show you where it is." After she led him into the house, the man grabbed a kitchen knife, robbed her and stabbed her several times. He then found a second knife and continued stabbing her until she died. Sometime during this ordeal the woman was also stripped and raped.

The killer was executed for this crime in 1990. Brutal to the end, his last words before being strapped to the electric chair were, "She should have locked her damn door."

Confronted with thousands of criminal and terrorist crimes, all preceded with, "May I use your telephone," one cannot help but wonder why we have allowed this one simple tactic to destroy so many lives.

"May I use your telephone" even launched the most highly publicized political kidnapping in U.S. history. On February 5, 1974, a woman came to the door of a Berkeley, California, apartment occupied by Patricia Hearst, nineteen, granddaughter to the late newspaper publisher William Randolph Hearst. The woman asked to use the telephone because her car had broken down. As the woman stepped inside she was followed by two men. Suddenly, the two men and the woman pulled weapons, beat Miss Hearst's fiancé, Stephen Weed, and dragged Patricia to a waiting car. In the biggest news event of the decade, Patricia Hearst had been kidnapped by the Symbionese Liberation Army (SLA). The rest is history.

REDUCING THE RISK

1. Face up to the fact and brief your children and baby-sitters that in the real world hundreds of criminals (thieves, sex offenders, serial murderers, and others) have utilized the "May I use your telephone" tactic. Many of these criminals are masters of deception and fully capable of telling sad, convincing stories.

2. The good news is that most people are not criminals. Therefore, if someone says, "There's been an accident and I need to call an ambulance" or "My car is broken down, I need to call a tow truck," have that person wait outside, keep the door locked and *you* call the ambulance or mechanic for them.

3. Your door should have a viewer (peephole) and/or intercom combination so that you can see and listen without opening the door. Remember, hundreds of times each year in the United States criminals "push in" once they get someone to open the door even a little. Many people utilize a chain on their door that allows the door to be opened a little but not so far that a criminal can squeeze in. Warning: If you use a chain make sure it is strongly secured; most chains pop easily from the frame when a criminal puts his shoulder to the door.

4. In many cases burglars (posing as workmen, real estate agents, etc.) ask to use the phone so that they can study the inside of your house or unlatch a window for later entry. In many cases people asking for the phone steal items laying about.

5. Criminals utilize many tricks. A rapist feigning an emergency smeared fake blood on his face and asked to call an ambulance; a burglar asking to call a tow truck carried jumper cables over his shoulder as a prop; a group of Gypsies robbing homes were having children "call their mothers." Once inside, the children were to (a) steal what they could get their hands on, (b) distract the homeowners while the older thieves entered a back door, and (c) unlock back doors and windows for later use.

6. Many women practice good security when they are alone but throw caution to the wind when they are not alone. It's true that there is sometimes "safety in numbers" but in most cases more people simply means more victims. There are literally hundreds of cases in which one or more gunmen brutalized an entire family and left men, women, and children injured or dead. Prevention is the best security. If you practice one security policy when you are alone, practice the same policy when other people are present.

7. Remember, criminals asking to use the phone have committed rape, robbery, murder, and kidnappings. They have surveilled home interiors, sized up defenses, placed listening devices, stolen keys (which were used at a later date), molested children, and so forth. The threat is real.

8. Criminals are increasingly female and there are many cases in which female criminals have asked, "May I use your telephone?" Don't underestimate the female criminal; she is as lethal as the male. In addition, many criminals utilizing this tactic have shown up at the front door posing as man and wife.

9. Criminals frequently exploit your charitable feelings during the Christmas season and criminals are frequently your neighbors! One Chicago woman didn't know her neighbor very well but allowed him to make an "important" phone call; after all, it was Christmas. She had no way of knowing that the man was a drug addict and was using this ruse to steal valuables. Caught in the act of stealing gifts from beneath the Christmas tree, he stabbed her to death. She was found next to the Christmas tree by her young daughter.

15
Workmen

A Virginia man was arrested by the police. He had posed as a maintenance worker and a plumber. He is suspected of committing more than two dozen rapes and robberies in the Washington area, attacking women ages seventeen to eighty-two years old in their apartments. Almost all of his attacks occurred in the daytime. He wore dark maintenance-type clothing. Sometimes he said he needed to check an air vent filter and sometimes he said he needed to check a leak in a water pipe. After telling one woman he needed to check her vent filter, he grabbed her from behind, forced her to a bed, and sexually assaulted her. Like many other criminals who have posed as workmen, this man used his work props (screwdriver, carpet knives, hammers) as weapons. And like many other fake workmen, he has a long history of utilizing this tactic. He had previously been sent to prison for posing as a plumber and robbing women in their homes. And, one year after being released from prison, he was convicted of raping another woman after pretending to be a building inspector. When a criminal finds a tactic that works, he usually sticks with it.

Scores of women have unwittingly assisted rapists and robbers by giving out too much information on the phone. If you insinuate that you live alone, a rapist will certainly take note. If you say you work the night shift as a nurse, a burglar will know when your apartment is empty. And if he has any doubt that you are away from your home, he simply calls you at the hospital. Even seemingly insignificant information can be valuable to a crook. One woman, apologizing for the static on her telephone, told a solicitor that "the whole building is having telephone problems." Women were not in the least bit suspicious when the solicitor, a full-time criminal, entered two apartments posing as a telephone repairman.

The phony workman, who has probably committed 200 crimes, is in jail today because one woman, suspicious of his activities, jotted down his license tag number. This woman probably doesn't realize it, but she has just prevented a few dozen rapes and robberies.

More than 100 crimes are committed against women every single day in the United States by men pretending to be plumbers, driveway repairmen, electricians, maintenance men, roofers, painters, building inspectors, and so forth. Pretending to be workmen, criminals commit over 36,500 crimes against women every year, in the home and office, and at least 80 percent of these crimes are absolutely preventable.

Sometimes a "plumber" will ask a resident to monitor an upstairs bathroom while he shuts the water off. "Is it off or on?" he will holler. Of course, while the woman is sequestered in the bathroom the plumber is plundering the rest of the house. One bogus workman was finally arrested May 15, 1992, in New York after terrorizing dozens of elderly women and men. Wearing a plumber's uniform, he would send the victim into the bathroom to run the water. While they were gone, he would rifle the rooms. Sometimes when he got caught, he would get violent. In one incident he dropped a toy gun while scuffling with an eighty-nine-year-old woman. The woman picked up the gun, pointed it at "the workman's" head, and pulled the trigger. She was disappointed to discover the weapon was a toy.

Sometimes the workmen work in pairs. While one man distracts the homeowner, a second man goes room to room, stealing. And sometimes the "workman" unlocks a basement window, steals a set of keys, or jams a door lock so that he can come back later.

Dozens of different cons are perpetrated, often against women, by phony workers. One scam is called the "concrete repair con." The resident, most commonly an elderly woman, is told that a relative or "the city" sent them to repair dangerous cracks in her driveway. The workers say they need buckets of hot water for the work. While one of the "workers" is in the basement running the water and engaging the woman in conversation, the other is looking for valuables in other parts of the house.

Then there's the "utility impostor scheme," where the scam artist tells homeowners that they have a rebate coming and asks them for change for a fifty-dollar bill. When the victim goes to get the change, the criminals note the hiding place. An accomplice later distracts the victim so that another member of the group can steal the victim's money.

In suburban Illinois, an elderly woman answered the doorbell and found two men at her door. The men said that the landlord asked them to check her windows for "seepage." While one man headed for the kitchen and talked loudly, the other man dashed for the bedroom. After the men departed, the woman discovered that thousands of dollars worth of jewelry was missing from her dresser drawers.

In many cases women have been attacked or swindled by criminals claiming to represent the water company. New York police arrested a man posing as a water meter reader. He forced nearly thirty women to pay him hundreds of dollars each. Claiming to be with the water company and using a computer printout as a prop, he told these women they owed two to five hundred dollars on their water bills. "I have to shut your water off, ma'am." Inching his way into the home, the man would show a phony bill and tell the women to pay cash now or it could be a long time before the water would be turned on again. This was the fourth time this criminal was arrested on similar charges.

Actually, several types of criminals, including serial rapists, have pretended to be with the water company. Police in Houston, Texas, arrested one man and linked him to fourteen rapes and a long series of burglaries, robberies, and assaults. Donning a white hard hat and carrying a clipboard, he had gained access to several women's homes by claiming to be a water tester.

Scores of women have been attacked in offices and apartment complexes by phony painters. In Silver Spring, Maryland, a woman allowed two men into her apartment when they told her they were painters. One of the men raped the woman. Afterward, the men stole a television, jewelry, and cash from the apartment. In most of the cases in which criminals posed as painters, the men carried buckets and brushes and dressed in paint-splattered overalls. Apparently, many of these impostors have an excellent gift of gab because the victims include several very sophisticated, well-educated women. Perhaps the "painters" just timed their attacks when the women, for some reason, had let their guard down. One woman told the author, "How could I have been so stupid!" Though it was of no consolation, she was in good company.

But women are not only being targeted by fake workmen. Women are also being attacked by real workmen hired to do jobs in the home and office.

A Texas woman was found dead in her bathtub. A fired maintenance worker at the victim's apartment complex was convicted of the crime. In Washington, D.C., a moving man was part of a crew that carried furniture at an unsuspecting woman's house. A week later, he returned to the home, broke into the basement, and murdered the woman and her daughter. In Illinois, a man was hired to paint the inside of a luxurious home. Shortly after being paid, he returned to the home, while the husband was on a fishing trip, and tortured and murdered the wife. She was raped, beaten, doused with gasoline, and then set afire. Badly burned, she managed to crawl to her front driveway but died a short time later.

Three women in Virginia were all raped by a repairman for a major retailer who came to their homes to repair appliances, and then returned later through a bedroom window or basement door. In each case, he used his job to find his victims, study their homes, and determine when they would be alone.

One of his victims returned to her home at night following a shopping trip. As she walked into her bedroom, the man, who had been waiting, reached out and grabbed her from behind. Quoted in the newspaper the victim said, "I screamed, but that wasn't very effective. He told me to shut up or he'd kill me." The woman did not recognize the rapist as the "very professional, competent, almost fatherly" repairman who had come to fix her air conditioner and check her furnace four weeks earlier. "It doesn't seem like there's any safe place anymore," said the victim. "I've always taken reasonable precautions. But the house wasn't safe."

Workmen, of course, are no more likely to commit crimes than any other profession. But like any profession, they have their bad apples, their bad 5 percent. The problem is that this 5 percent has access to your home and office.

In recent years, there have been at least twenty cases in which carpet cleaners have committed murders, rapes, robberies, and even offenses against children. During June 1991 in Gainesville, Florida, a man hired to clean carpets in student apartments strangled two young women to death. He was convicted of killing the two students. He said one of the women made a pass at him and then for some reason sprayed him with Mace. He said he punched her and strangled her to death. When the other woman came to her roommate's aid, he strangled her, too.

Parents who had hired a Virginia carpet-cleaning company were appalled to learn that the owner had abducted an eight-year-old girl. He had dragged the little girl into his van, forced her to perform oral sex, and then raped her. The carpet cleaner, who has worked in many homes with children, has been convicted and incarcerated.

A woman interviewed by the author, who was raped in her office building by a janitor, was both "sick and furious" to learn that the man had two prior rape convictions, both incidents occurring in an office building. The janitor, who had been drinking, attacked the woman while she was working alone, at about seven P.M., when most of her co-workers had gone home.

Unfortunately, scores of women have been attacked in the workplace by workmen and professionals alike.

A woman was stabbed to death by a janitor in a Washington, D.C., office building. In planning the robbery, the janitor reportedly told a co-worker that if the victim resisted, he would kill her. In Florida, a janitor stabbed and killed a young woman as she worked late at her office. Both incidents occurred within a couple of days of Christmas.

Increasingly, women are learning that they are not only threatened by criminals posing as workmen but also by legitimate employees, both blue collar and white collar, hired to work in their homes, apartment complexes, and offices.

REDUCING THE RISK

1. Remember, criminals posing as painters, plumbers, maintenance men, roofers, electricians, meter readers, building inspectors, and so forth victimize more than 100 women every day in the United States.

2. Be very suspicious of workmen who appear at your door unannounced. Keep the door locked and do not invite the workmen in until you are confident the situation is legitimate. Verify their authenticity by checking their identification and calling their office. Do not be fooled by props and official-looking documents.

3. Take control of the situation. Don't let one workman distract you while his partner roams the house. Be suspicious and cautious if a plumber or electrician asks you to monitor the water or electricity in another room.

4. Get involved in security. If you have reason to be suspicious of workmen in your apartment complex, report your concerns to the management.

5. You are most vulnerable when you are alone. If a workman is going to be present in your home, ask a friend to keep you company. This reduces the threat to you and the friend can help monitor the workman.

6. Protect your keys! In hundreds of cases, workmen have stolen keys. In Maryland, a part-time handyman stole house keys, apparently when he entered the house to use the bathroom. He returned later and murdered a young woman in her sleep.

   If you have had workmen in your home for an extended period of time, it might be wise to change your locks. Are you missing any keys?

7. Always ask to be billed! Be very suspicious of anyone asking you for cash.

8. Be aware of the "stay behind" tactic so frequently used by criminals in offices. They come in as workers during normal working hours and then just before closing hide in closets, rest rooms, ceilings, etc. When everyone has gone home the "worker" comes out of hiding. Several women have been raped by "stay behind" criminals.

9. Always think security! Thousands of women have been raped, robbed, or murdered by criminals posing as workmen. Thousands more have been attacked in the home and office by legitimate workmen. These are the facts. You must always think survival.